Peyton Quinn

Author of *A Bound...*

R

FIGHTING

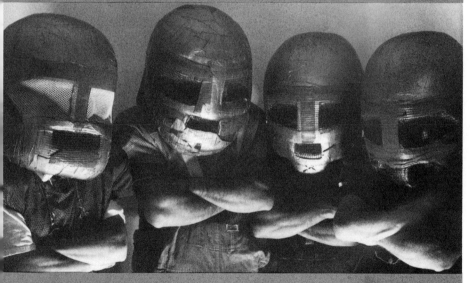

Adrenaline Stress Conditioning through Scenario-Based Training

Paladin Press • Boulder, Colorado

Other Books and Videos by Peyton Quinn:

A Bouncer's Guide to Barroom Brawling: Dealing with
the Sucker Puncher, Streetfighter, and Ambusher

Barroom Brawling: The Art of Staying Alive in
Beer Joints, Biker Bars, and Other Fun Places (video)

Black Medicine: The Video

Blitzkrieg Attacks: Knockout Blows
from the Bouncer Trade (video)

Defending against the Blade (video)

Self-Defense against the Sucker Puncher (video)

Real Fighting:
Adrenaline Stress Conditioning through Scenario-Based Training
by Peyton Quinn

Copyright © 1996 by Peyton Quinn

ISBN 0-87364-893-5
Printed in the United States of America

Published by Paladin Press, a division of
Paladin Enterprises, Inc., P.O. Box 1307,
Boulder, Colorado 80306, USA.
(303) 443-7250

Direct inquiries and/or orders to the above address.

Contents

Adrenal Stress-Based Learning Stays with the Individual Forever
Why Traditional Martial Arts Training Is Incomplete Preparation for an
Actual Self-Defense Encounter

Classical Martial Arts as "Ancient and Proven Combat Systems"
The Uncommon Quality of Common Sense
Are There Really "True Masters?"
What Makes a Master?
Very Few Real Fights Are Decided by Subtle or Master Technique
What the Scenario Training Method Achieves
Scenario Training Works for Both Black Belts and Untrained Fighters

A Pistol You Don't Have with You Won't Help
One Learns to Fight Empty-Handed Because Most Times,
"That's All You Got"
Scenario Training Should Be Mandatory for Police
There Is Just as Much Misinformation in Firearms Training as
There Is in the Martial Arts World
An Exception: Jeff Cooper's Principles of Personal Defense
The Problem with Experience and Dogmatism
An Experiment In Adapting Scenario-Based Training to the
Combat Use of the Pistol
Some Observations about Our Scenario-Based Pistol Training
The Primary Goal of Scenario Training with Weapons:
Developing The Proper Mind-Set
Extraordinary Martial Skill with the Weapon Is Not Demanded to
Survive Most Real-World Attacks
Scenario Training Using the Stick
The Dog Brothers
A Final Note: The Most Dangerous Assailants Don't Display Their
Weapons before Using Them

Proper Response to Adrenal Stress Can Be Learned
All Cruelty Comes from Weakness

Preface

AN IMPORTANT LESSON IN COMBAT ATTITUDE

When I was a kid, maybe 13 years old, I'd save my pennies and buy any book in print on martial arts. I would study the black and white photographs in detail and read and reread every word of them. They promised much: "Instantly render any assailant helpless" or "For the first time, the Deadly Monkey Hands of Steel are revealed by Master Chang Lee Dang," and so on, ad nauseam.

They promised much, but none of these books really seemed to help.

Even at the tender age of 13, I'd been in more than a few scraps, and the stuff I saw in those books either seemed too obvious, too unrealistic for a real battle, or just incomprehensible altogether.

My father's work had moved us from state to state, and I was enrolled in one school after another. Without fail, each new school came complete with its own class bully, and the bully's first duty always seemed to be to "test the new kid."

This shit got old, like real fast. I didn't like being pushed around, and I just wasn't going to take it.

Physically, however, I was still a kid barely on the threshold of puberty, while my enemies had always been "held back" a grade or two. This meant that the bullies were literally twice my size and thus seemingly impossible opponents to overcome.

Still, I had to find a way to deal with them. Hence, my interest (a masterpiece of understatement) in martial arts, particularly the Asian systems.

Then an incident occurred that instructed me both tactically and spiritually concerning the reality of personal combat and what it truly meant to overcome a "stronger" enemy. Most importantly of all, it would teach me the critical significance of *attitude* in determining victory or defeat.

It was in a small-town junior high school that this lesson was presented to me, but it was certainly no intentional part of that institution's curriculum. My teacher was to be the greatest instructor of all in "life's realities," which is simply life itself. This perfect instructor showed me the perfect truth of my dilemma: the person I had to overcome was not the new bully at all, but *myself!*

ENTER THE "CARROT TOP"

Act One of this little drama played itself out while I was waiting in the lunch line at the new school. A very large person with carrot-red hair approached me and demanded 10 cents of my lunch money. The school lunch in those days cost 25 cents.

I had one quarter and one dime—35 cents total. That extra dime was destined for the purchase of an ice cream sandwich as far as I was concerned. My nemesis had other ideas and informed me that in exchange for the dime, and an equal payment each succeeding day, he would not break my arm.

This deal seemed a bit one-sided to me, and I informed him that, "For 10 cents you can kiss the sweat off my balls." A bold statement, indeed, especially since, at the time, those young testicles were not even fully descended.

My lunch-line bravado was partially the result of my expectation that he wouldn't be ready to make his move and stomp me right then and there, since "adult" guards were present. It certainly was not based on any idea that I could possibly represent any physical challenge to him. After all, had I not looked up when standing "face to face" with this dude, my eyes would have been staring at a spot just above his navel.

As I'd anticipated, the battle did not go down right then and there, but before the lunch period was over I became aware of the true scope and consequences of my defiance. The individual who had attempted to extort my lunch money was the leader of the second most powerful gang in the school, and it was now common knowledge that he and his associates were going to stomp my ass as soon as I left the safety of the lunchroom.

Although I remember the person's name clearly (even after the intervening 30-plus years), I'll just call him "Carrot Top."

My first defense strategy against being beaten senseless by Carrot Top as soon as I left the safety of the lunchroom was simply not to leave the safety of the lunchroom. Unfortunately, this simple plan was complicated somewhat by the fact that the adult guards forced everybody out of the lunchroom once they had finished eating.

My solution to this problem was to go directly from the lunchroom to the lavatory, where I hung out a bit until no one else was there. At that point, standing on the window sill, I was just able to push up one of the suspended ceiling panels and pull my skinny 80-pound body up into the space between the ceiling and the roof. I then slipped the ceiling panel back in place.

Inside this dark sanctuary, I waited until I heard the passing bell ring and then quickly dropped back down before anyone could get back into the lavatory.

This strategy was repeated the next day . . . and the day after that.

I was terrified of the beating I knew I'd receive at Carrot Top's hands, and anything seemed preferable to that unknown horror. I'd gotten black eyes and bloody noses before dealing with other bully types, but Carrot Top was a different deal for sure. This guy was enormous; he must have outweighed me by at least my total body weight. On top of all this, he'd have his boys with him. There seemed to be "no way out."

I'd lie in bed at night and imagine all the different types of painful, even permanently disabling injuries that could result from my being stomped by Carrot Top and his crew.

At this point my fear controlled me completely. This was intolerable. And so I refused to tolerate it.

As I was lying there in bed, my mind went through a remarkable series of transformations. It began when I decided that I could not hide out forever, and even if I could, I was no longer willing to do so.

The next thought I had was, "How bad am I really likely to be hurt?"

Once I thought about it, all I really knew was that Carrot Top and his boys had broken one kid's arm; administered multiple burns to another kid's face with their cigarettes; and bruised, bloodied, and knocked down a few others. While none of this seemed too pleasant, nobody had actually been killed or crippled. Once I really faced it, my worst fear wasn't really as terrible as my own imagination had portrayed it.

"So, okay," I thought, "I'll get the shit stomped out of me, and then Carrot Top will be satisfied and it will all be over with.

That's what I really was looking for, too—just a way to get it all over with. Even a brutal beating was infinitely preferable to the daily fear and hiding I had been experiencing.

Next, I thought, "How, exactly, is this beating likely going to take place?"

I'd dealt with bullies before, and in my mind's eye I played back the images of how I'd seen them operate in the past. It occurred to me that very often before beating somebody up they would direct some grievance or verbal declaration of intent toward the victim before the festivities actually began. Even then I knew that these brief little speeches by the bully were really not meant for the victim but to impress the bully's own entourage and intimidate the general populace.

After the words usually came the shove, a punch, a takedown, and then the kicking and stomping would begin. Once the victim hit the ground, and never before, other members of the bully's gang would participate in the stomping.

What the hell? Since I knew this would likely be the pattern, I thought, why not get just one shot in before I got stomped? I'd have to jump up in the air to reach Carrot Top's face, but I figured this was possible.

My objective was to make a symbolic gesture, mostly to make me feel better about the whole deal. Still, I wanted to maximize my chances of landing that one symbolic shot, and so I thought, "What would be the best way to achieve this? And when would be the best time?"

As I pondered this logically, it first occurred to me that the best time to throw my punch would be when he gathered his troops around and came real close to me to make that anticipated little speech before actually shoving me off my feet. I knew he wouldn't be expecting anything, since he was completely confident that I could not possibly represent any threat to him whatsoever.

I continued this line of thinking. Having decided when to make my move, the next question became, how I could best insure my being able to get that one shot in before I went down? And then, how could I best make that shot worth something—maybe actually causing the bastard some pain, or at least momentary embarrassment?

Later that night, the final plan came to me in all its

audacious splendor. Before I had turned off the light to go to bed that night, my mind had been in turmoil, dominated by fear, but now, I was actually beginning to feel pretty good. I was very much aware that all that had changed as I lay there thinking was simply my attitude. I had "gotten my mind right."

FIRST BLOOD: THE CREEPY CRIMSON MAKES ITS APPEARANCE

The next day as I waited in the lunch line, I subtly let others cut in front of me as I watched and counted the lunch trays popping up from the spring-loaded carrier. Most trays were plastic, but some were made of metal. I timed my arrival at the tray station to make sure I got a metal one.

After I got my tray, I shuffled past Carrot Top's table, where he sat every day, right there on the aisle. He sat with his gang members in that seat at "his" table, so he could occasionally amuse himself by tripping people carrying their trays of food as they passed by.

I was completely calm as I walked past Carrot Top, who was sitting down at the lunch table just like I'd planned. His being seated had equalized his height advantage, since I was walking and standing. Our heads were now at just about the same level.

He began to turn his head around toward me, likely to call out some challenge, threat, or insult just as I passed by. That made it perfect.

I instantly dumped the contents of the tray on the floor and, holding it with both hands, spun around and whacked it squarely into Carrot Top's face with everything I had. I swung the aluminum tray like a baseball bat with good, relaxed hip rotation and power, and it felt real good.

To my amazement, he did not jump up immediately and begin stomping me.

Indeed, after a fraction of a second of delay at this new wonderment, I realized he was really stunned. He was holding his hand out in front of him, looking with astonishment at the small amount of blood that had come from his nose. In that next millisecond, I stepped back for a bit more leverage and slammed the tray even more forcefully into his face.

As the followers of Islam are fond of saying, "*Allah Akhbar!,*" which simply means, "God is Great!"

Upon the second shot, Carrot Top was knocked out of his chair onto the floor. I jumped on top of him at once and began delivering a quick and repetitive series of whacks into his cranium with the metal tray. The dude was now bleeding like a Kushite bush pig, and I was beginning to experiment with blows to his head using the edge of the tray instead of the flat part when several adults finally pulled me off the guy. It was just like Christmas.

THE POINT OF THIS SCHOOLBOY TALE

Previously, I said that this had been a very instructive lesson for me, both tactically and spiritually. Yet some of you might be saying, "Sounds great. Now, if I can just get my enemies to sit down in a chair while I rustle up a metal food tray and ambush them, I'm in business!"

Glad to hear it—shows you're paying attention and thinking pragmatically.

While I could go so far as to say that every important lesson about overcoming the enemy is demonstrated in this simple schoolboy tale, I'll spare you this for the moment and draw your attention only to a few very important elements.

The metal tray helped a lot, of course. But would the tray alone have been of any value had I not first gotten my mind right? The correct answer is no. In fact, that tray would have remained in the tray dispenser and never would have found its way into my hands in the first place.

Extending this argument, do you see that even a pistol is of no use to you in a fight if haven't got your mind right?

In the same manner, martial arts techniques, of whatever style or to whatever level of proficiency they may have been developed, will also be of no value without "proper mind." Many martial artists discover this when they face their first real confrontation. Like the metal lunch tray that could have remained in the dispenser, their techniques and "skills" remain in the dojo.

Conversely, with proper mind, and in the absence of any knowledge of fighting techniques, you have a much better chance against the enemy than if you were accomplished at martial techniques but were not psychologically prepared for combat.

GETTING DOWN TO CASES

The following are some other things you need to appreciate about this incident because they represent specific applications of fundamental concepts in combat tactics and strategy:

(1) *I decided the time and place for the battle and did not let my enemy do so.* Keep this in mind the next time somebody challenges you to "step outside and settle it." Mainly, do not accept the invitation. Never let your enemy choose the time or place of the battle if you can avoid it.

(2) *I made use of my environment and what was at hand*—in this case, the metal tray. It is rare that you will have to battle an enemy where there exists no weapon potential. If nothing else, the walls and floors can be effective weapons if you know how to use them. Therefore, we are going to take a look at this idea of the environment as a weapon.

(3) *Since I took the initiative with the attack, I caused my enemy to "choke" and did not hesitate.* Carrot Top was not knocked unconscious by that first blow; he was simply stunned, that is, his mind was stopped for a moment when he felt the pain and saw his own blood, maybe for the first time. In short, *he choked!* I attacked him immediately and

continuously! If you can make your enemy choke and then press the attack relentlessly, never giving him a chance to come back, then victory is yours.

(4) *When I attacked, I was not thinking of anything else* but impacting that tray against Carrot Top's face. There was no "divided mind"; that is, there was no part of myself holding back any other part of me from fear of being hurt or for any other reason. My mind was relaxed, my mind was one, and it was resolute. In my mind, the tray had already struck my enemy's head before I'd swung that first blow.

GETTING YOUR MIND RIGHT

I have said that contained within this childhood battle are most, maybe all, of the important lessons in personal combat. Observe how each one of the items I listed above turns *principally* on correct attitude rather than on a particular physical skill.

A big part of "proper mind" is a relaxed mind. In principle #4 above, I am referring to the effect that a relaxed mind has on the execution of technique. One way to say this is, "Don't think about it; just step up and do it!"

Being of such "one mind" is a powerful thing and must be experienced to be appreciated fully. Perhaps it was best phrased by the samurai Musashi about 400 years ago: "Think neither of victory nor of yourself, but only of cutting and killing your enemy."

Whether it is with swords, guns, or even air-to-air heat-seeking missiles fired from supersonic jets, a fight is still a fight. The most decisive element will often be the mind-set of the combatants rather than their weapons, "technical skill," or anything else.

CHAPTER ONE

Perfect Intent Is More Important than Perfect Technique

IT'S ALWAYS LATER THAN YOU THINK

At some point in their lives people make fundamental decisions about their personal natures and their personal destinies. If they do not make such decisions, most often they simply drift through life, and things "happen to them" rather than their "making things happen."

Ironically, because of its extreme brevity, all of life's big changes rush upon us, one right after the other.

In my own case, it was fairly early in my life that circumstances and events made clear to me the fragility of the life experience . . . its brevity, its horror, and its sublime beauty. The personal decision that came to me was that I was not destined for, nor would I be content with, what may be called the "ordinary life."

Consequently, since that schoolboy encounter with "Carrot Top" so many years ago, I have faced a number of hand-to-hand battles with various assailants. Some were armed with only fists or bottles, others with pool cues, a few with knives, and one with a firearm. As a result, I have taken more than a few punches that made me see those whitish-purple stars against that black background. I've been cut up with blades a bit, and I had a slug penetrate my tender flesh. In short, I've had more than my share of luck, because I wasn't killed, or worse. (Keep in mind that as far as luck is concerned, just being born in any one of these United States—except New Jersey, of course—is a cosmic break from Jump Street on a global scale and of epic proportions.)

However, since you did not purchase this book to endure my personal memoirs, and having indulged myself to this extent, I'll get on with it.

But before I do, let me say that it will demand some serious attention on your part if you want to get some real, practical, and applied self-defense benefit out of this information. You are investing your time in reading this book. I hope that you will try to absorb its full content. I do not think this will be achieved by only a light reading; it will require study and some attention. You must also find training partners to explore these concepts and practice the techniques with.

SOME VERY IMPORTANT COMBAT CONCEPTS

In my first book, *A Bouncer's Guide to Barroom Brawling*, I spent a lot of time describing why fights occur, the psychology of the bully, his techniques, and his methods for selecting prey. An understanding of these things is necessary to actualize a personal awareness and avoidance strategy that will help you avoid most of these distressed and dangerous people in the first place.

I reiterate, recognizing and avoiding these people is the real art. Once you are forced to fight, your awareness/avoidance strategy has already failed, and anything can happen.

Not every potential fight can be avoided, I admit, but keep in mind that I have seen hundreds of fights, and I will tell you that most could have been avoided if handled properly. This was one of the central themes of my first book: "*A fight avoided is a fight won.*" Also in that first book I put forth the central methods and physical techniques I used as a bouncer to avoid having my teeth knocked out or being fatally sliced up during that time in my life. I did so in part because they were easy *techniques* to learn and I had used them habitually to defeat the most common attacks. But I also presented them as vehicles to convey the following fundamental combat *concepts*:

(1) relaxation
(2) not contesting the enemy's power
(3) continuous attack

For those readers who have not read my first book, let me give some brief explanations of these three fundamental combat concepts.

Relaxation: Imagine someone concentrating on a book in a quiet library and someone else accidentaly drops a book to the floor with a loud "bang." Many people reading who hear the sound will "tense" their muscles involuntarily.

When we expect to be hit or are face to face with a menacing bully, is it is also natural to tense up. But this handicaps our defense greatly because we cannot move quickly; we are fighting the tension in our own muscles put there by a mind that is not relaxed. If we can keep a more calm and relaxed mind we can move faster and more precisely and fluidly.

Not contesting the enemy's power: In a very important sense if you are relaxed in your mind, then already you are not contesting the enemy's power. The most fundamental expression of this concept is slipping a blow rather than blocking it. When we slip a blow it slides past us and its power is not contested. When we block a blow we are almost directly contesting the enemy's power. You cannot block a machete strike with your naked arm, nor can you block a much stronger man's punch this way. But you *can* slip the machete blow or the stronger man's punch. This is not contesting the enemy's power.

Continuous attack: Take the fight to the enemy. Never pause to judge the effectiveness of a blow you have just landed. This is a critical error; you must attack continiously. Once you have struck your enemy you must continue with one strike after another relentlessly. You must never give the enemy the chance to recover and to defend himself.

When you truly understand what these concepts mean and internalize them, you will begin the actualization of your own martial potential. To internalize something means to make it part of you, not on a superconscious level, but reflexively, like when your hand hits a hot stove and you jerk it away. Many persons study martial arts for many years without achieving this understanding, so I will not pretend it's easy, but it is necessary.

In this chapter we'll examine in further depth the fundamental concept of relaxation and how essential it is to successful self-defense.

THE FEAR FACTOR

For most people, the biggest problem they face in defending themselves effectively is simply dealing properly with their fear. When people are unable to control their fear, they cannot *relax,* even under the threat of an attack, much less during the attack itself. Their attackers perceive this during the initial "interview" (discussed at length in *Bouncer's Guide to Barroom Brawling* and below) and are thus encouraged to attack.

DYNAMIC RELAXATION

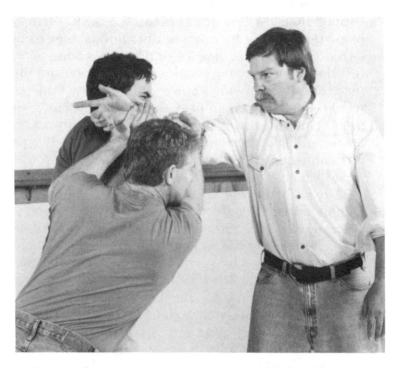

There is nothing mystical going on here in my way of thinking. It is an exercise that most anyone can be taught how to do in a matter of a few minutes. It is popular in aikido training, where it is called "unbendable arm." The two individuals are using all the force they can muster to bend my arm, but my arm remains straight while my hand is open and my arm "relaxed" in an important sense. This is also an example of not contesting power.

While this exercise can be seen as just another "parlor trick" suitable primarily for the glossy covers of martial arts magazines, I submit that it has some practical value as well. When people discover that they can do this, then they are experiencing "dynamic relaxation" and thus know what it feels like. This also shows them in a tangible, nonmetaphysical way that mind controls body.

When teaching a given self-defense technique, I might see someone who is either too tensed up (or, conversely, too limp) in his arms as he rehearses the given self-defense technique. If he has experienced the immovable arm exercise earlier, I can then simply grab his limb while he is practicing with his training partner and say something like, "Relax it, this is the immovable arm," and they know what I mean and can do the technique more properly.

When the assault does come, fear/rage tenses the victims' minds and their muscles; thus, they have handicapped their own defense potential dramatically. Not being relaxed (but focused) in their minds, they cannot be relaxed in their bodies. Their limbs thus tense to meet the blows, even in expectation of the blows, and thus, they contest the enemy's power. It is all part of the same whole: expecting the impact, they receive same. I, your humble narrator, as well as any of my ex-bouncer buddies—the Eagle, the Mad Chinaman—have seen this phenomenon many times in our bar work, and occasionally we have seen a good simulation of it even in the dojo.

The reality of the disabling effects of fear has been demonstrated to me further at our training program in Colorado, where we simulate with fidelity all the essential elements of a real challenge and a real attack. Even in these simulations I have seen many people—even black belts—"choke" the first time out. However, after several of these simulations, it's like they are different people; they blast with beauty, they slam, and they grind. Their blows have proper timing and carry the necessary juice. It's a wonderment to behold, because they have transcended their fear!

Just as in my schoolboy tale in the Introduction, all that has really changed with these people is their attitude! Mind truly controls body!

It is my sincere belief that most people can learn to defend themselves to a reasonable degree once they get their minds right. Conversely, no amount of training or fighting "skill" is going to be of much use in a real attack if you have not begun to control your fear and thus control your body under adrenal stress.

An Example of Having One's Mind Right

Consider the housewife who may have given no real thought at all to ever having to deal with physical violence (denial) and is then confronted with a rapist. She may choke and submit. Perhaps she has decided that this is her best survival strategy under the specific circumstances.

But then the rapist, having finished with her, goes into her child's room. Suddenly, the rapist ends up with a pair of scissors stuck through the back of his neck . . . repeatedly. This woman would be an example of someone getting her mind right once she became properly motivated.

Amazing to me, yet an observable reality that cannot be dismissed, is that some people are not properly motivated to defend themselves because of a weak self-image or lack of self-esteem. In effect (perhaps even at the subconscious level), they have some feeling that they may not be worth fighting for.

Search your own heart and mind, and if any such thoughts exist there, *purge them.*

You *are* worth fighting for!

The Essential Cowardice of the Bully

Just like the barroom bully or sucker puncher, the rapist was counting on his victim being paralyzed with fear, which he expected would prevent her from offering any effective resistance.

The rapist, a diseased life form, is just a particular version of every bully. They are all looking for an easy victim because, generally, they don't want to risk being hurt themselves. This is also why immediate, determined, and forceful resistance will many times drive off rapists. They are true cowards. This doesn't mean that they can't kill you—they may—but I am convinced from my own experience that most every bully is the coward, constantly in fear that he will be found out.

The Bully Often Retreats in the Face of a Relaxed Mind

The psychology of the bully should illuminate for you the reality that it is *how you respond to the bully's probing and interviewing techniques* (either verbally or nonverbally) that will most often determine whether he will actually attack you. He is searching for the signs in your face and in your actions and spirit that to him say, "Weak or uncertain self-image—this one's going to be safe to attack."

With a few students in our training programs, one of the central things we do is to incrementally increase their feelings of self-worth and self-confidence so that they can overcome their fear and then blast and crack righteously upon their assailant. Having done this and thus having successfully realized their power, their self-confidence is elevated even further. This means they have made themselves much less attractive victims for the bully in his research for easy prey.

The same fundamental combat concepts have been articulated in different ways and in different tongues throughout history by many people who have had some acquaintance with battle. This is no accident. These things are repeated because they represent fundamental and significant truths about battle—any type of battle. Again, consider the woman who submitted to the rape but stabbed the assailant to death when he threatened her child. Consider her mind-set when she picked up those scissors and came up behind her enemy. She was thinking "neither of victory, nor of herself, but only of cutting and killing her enemy," just as the sword saint of Japan, Musashi, instructed 400 years previously. In the 16th century with a samurai's sword or in the 20th century with a housewife's pair of scissors, *it's the same*!

Some Interview Techniques You Should Be Aware of

The most common interview technique begins with the hard eyes from across the room. The potential victim may try to ignore it. This will elicit the next step in the bully or predator's program, which most often will be a "woof," such as, "What the fuck are you looking at, dickhead?!" If not derailed by the potential victim, this program will often culminate in a punch-out.

Sometimes the interviewer is not looking for a victim to punch out right then, just someone who is safe to humiliate verbally. Either way, it's the same interview process used to identify the safe victim. Be aware that verbal humiliation may just be an extended, long-term interview technique itself. In other words, it is only after having verbally humiliated someone over a period of time (a few days, a week, or several months) without any retaliation that the bully becomes confident that it is safe to attack physically.

Appreciate that there are several styles and types of interview techniques, but most are not too hard to spot—generally very early on—if you are just aware of them. An exception, and the most dangerous type of interview, is the one that occurs silently in the mind of the assailant as he surveys potential prey. This is the method of the basic psycho interviewer, and it seems the psycho interviewer more frequently attacks with the knife. Still, even this guy can be spotted if you are very alert (crazy eyes).

The briefer the interview, the more it resembles the straight ambush. But even the guy that just says, "Fuck you!" and throws the sucker punch is still using an interview technique, it's just that his is very economical and fast. The "fuck you" is still meant to make you freeze in order to facilitate the attack and summon the attacker's own "courage."

A classic ambush interview style that I experienced one night about a year or so ago in a Denver city parking lot might be called the "Got a Match/Got a Dollar?" In this interview/ambush variation the predator chooses a location for its absence of other persons except the intended victim. The predator will appear in front of you and ask for a match or maybe a dollar. Often, his appearance will be sudden and unexpected. His real objective is to draw your attention to himself in front of you so that his partner(s) can attack you from behind. Cro-Magnon man must have used this ambush technique.

If you doubt this stone-age ambush technique is an interview at all, consider my experience with it. I had been fortunate enough to have spotted the guy before I even crossed the street into the parking lot where my car was. When the "front man" appeared it was expected, and I stepped off the attack line and turned around immediately to stare right at the two guys behind me. After a little "crazy man, ready to die" act on my part, they gave up their intention to roll me without our ever having to do any physical fighting at all.

Their clear intention was to knock me down from behind and rob me of whatever I had on me. Their "Got a Match?" interview was designed to simply set up the pieces in the ideal positions for their little drama. But it was still an interview, and my behavior put me outside of their perception of someone safe to attack. After all, they knew all they had to do was be a little patient, and in a short while another potential victim would certainly show up.

The next, more protracted type of interview often occurs where alcohol is served. This interview technique can sometimes be more difficult to spot, because the person may not seem at all hostile initially. Popular topics of conversation for such predators include the Vietnam War, racial hatred, homosexuality, and, of course, politics in general. The way this works is the predator maneuvers you into a position in the conversation where he identifies you (rightly or not—after all, it's all happening in his mind) as the enemy: a "God-damn-faggot war protester," a "nigger lover," or simply a "faggot" or "commie." Now he is ready to either assault you or escalate his verbal humiliation to full intensity to force you to leave "his" space.

There are disturbed people who do this sort of thing habitually and don't even realize they are doing it. Obvious as it may seem, it bears repeating: normal, decent people, regardless of their race, sexuality, or politics, don't bully or assault other people. Because of this, the bully and the interview in this case are really not that hard to spot at all. The main reason they are not spotted as often as they could be is because the interview is always unpleasant, somewhat frightening, and bizarre. Therefore, the potential victim often denies the interview rather than facing it and dealing with it immediately. The interviewer counts on this pattern.

THE IDEAL COMBAT MIND-SET

The ideal combat mind-set is one of a focused but

relaxed mind that projects your own resolute spirit through the enemy's mind. In this state, you are in no hurry to get things done because you have "seen" your enemy's defeat before he throws his first shot. This cannot truly be explained in words.

However, this thought may one day provide you with the context necessary to appreciate a big part of why you prevail in some future confrontation. It really makes no difference whether you prevail by shutting down the interview and thus avoiding the attack altogether, or if the guy actually did attack and you blasted him and laid him out on the floor. The ideal mind-set for either activity is exactly the same on the most important level.

The Experience of Rage on the Path to Proper Mind

Many people's first experience on the road to developing proper fighting attitude is simply the emotion of rage. This rage may occur when someone threatens to beat them up or actually does hit them. At that point, they may just "go off" for the first time in their lives in pure outrage that someone would abuse them like that *and think he could get away with it!* Having thus gone off, they are momentarily possessed of abnormally great physical speed, strength, and tolerance to pain as adrenaline flows unchecked into their bloodstreams.

Well, all this is a good start.

It may even be that rage is a necessary stage in developing proper combat attitude. But I will point out that indignant rage is still another expression of fear, although it is a much more combat-functional expression than simply being "frozen" in terror.

Rage is blind; it preempts rational thought and abandons any knowledge of training and technique.

To underscore this point, consider a trained karateka who may be a black belt in his art but who (to his credit) has never been in a fight because it has never been forced upon him. One day, someone calls him out, points a finger at him, threatens to "kick his ass," and then closes distance to shove him back (and off balance) in prelude and preparation for throwing the punch.

During this "woofing stage," the karateka may experience denial momentarily. This occurs when a part of his mind is telling him, "This can't really be happening." This is understandable, because the karateka has never experienced this stuff before. He has never been exposed to the interview cues that precede an attack. Consequently, he doesn't recognize them and does not interpret them correctly. He fails to realize that *with the woof the attack has already begun.* Believe me, this happens plenty of times.

But then, in the next instant, another part of his brain feels the shove or the punch, and the inner voice screams out, "FUCK! THIS IS HAPPENING! ATTACK! KILL! DESTROY! . . . ARHHHH!"

Got the picture?

Very likely, after going off like this, the karate-trained person may beat the shit out of his aggressor. But guess what? To watch him fight, you would never guess that this "karate guy" had ever even heard of karate. He simply goes "animal" and, in his rage, forgets all concept of precision karate technique. He just whales and blasts.

Once again, though it is not ideal, there is something very functional and positive to be said for just going off in an animal rage. It is, for example, far better than the karateka or anyone else in the same situation either showing obvious fear, thus encouraging the attack, or simply being sucker-punched and knocked senseless right off the bat (because of a lack of awareness skills).

Avoidance is Always the Best Self-Defense Strategy

Finally, I can't leave this idea without pointing out that *if* you have the awareness level and spot the interviewer in the first place, *then* it will be only the failure of your *avoidance* strategies that puts you in jeopardy by getting you in a fight in the first place.

Therefore, you should study and practice your avoidance strategies at least as hard as you do your offensive techniques. I have attempted to communicate to you why developing the ability to show no fear and to relax under the threat is a critical part of your *avoidance strategy.*

Imagine how someone might interview you—what they might say to push your "hot buttons" or to make you choke or go into denial. Then, picture yourself seeing right through it right while it's all happening and being relaxed rather than reactive. You might even have one of your training partners woof on you, that is, threaten you or challenge you to fight with verbal abuse in a realistic manner, just so you can experience how it feels biochemically. If you try this, you must first agree there will be no physical contact. And if you and your partner do it realistically, even though you know the person who's woofing on you, I will bet you will be very much surprised at how much it gets to you.

You must first be in control of yourself before you can have any control over the situation itself. The predator's interview is designed to both test you and then deny you such control. The earlier you perceive that you are the object of such an interview in the real world, the easier it will all be for you.

The Karateka Who Fails to Enter the Fight

Now let's consider another example of what sometimes happens when a guy with significant martial arts training and supposed fighting skill meets his first real-world attack. In this case, we assume the martial artist is aware and relaxed enough to avoid the sucker punch from nowhere, get something on it, and move out of the way before he gets hit, thus buying himself that all-important chance to fight. (Understand that many—maybe most—martial artists never get this far in their first real fight because they are blind-sided and knocked senseless before they can do anything. The sucker puncher then continues to blast and the martial arts guy gets stomped before he has a chance to block a single strike or throw a single shot himself. Sadly, this is really the norm.) Now the fight is on, because the martial arts guy knows he is under attack. Unfortunately, if he's only had most types of dojo training, he does not know what a fight really is, and so he fails to "enter the fight" instantly, which is another way of saying he fails to close on his enemy. (This is more than just a physical "closing"; it has to do with his psychological preparedness to engage the enemy.) Such an individual will often jump back from his enemy, assume a karate stance, or maybe begin to dance about his enemy from a "safe distance," treating the actual attack like a karate sparring match (like in his dojo). The only difference is that now, he's hot and has got the intent of full contact. The karate guy who attempts to defend himself with such a mind-set will most often hit the pavement real hard and real fast against the common street fighter.

Melissa Soalt, a woman who, until recently, taught self-defense in Boston (and did a damn good job of it, too) as the founder and former owner of Boston Model Mugging, once articulated the essential quality the fighter must have to avoid this crippling mind-set as the ability "to go from zero to 100 percent instantly." It's hard for most people to make this big transition in mind-set the first time out in a real fight. To do so demands that one's mind instantly disengage from anything but the combat imperative of striking down the enemy directly. The obstacle to effecting this is often that some portion of the conscious or semiconscious mind is saying, "This isn't happening . . . in another moment I'll see that, I don't want to do this, I might get hurt, violence can be avoided."

This is why the term "denial" is used. There is a danger in slapping labels on things, but my experience tells me this one fits. Keep in mind that your enemy is counting on your momentary denial for his assured victory. When you mentally deny the reality of the attack (even the cues that precede it), you have hesitated and you have choked. Of course, all this is a two-way street. As I said earlier, if *you* can make your enemy choke, victory is yours.

Do you see that the karate dancer's way of dealing with the real fight like a dojo sparring match is another expression of denial? Having failed to enter the fight, he is struck down by the sucker puncher's continuous attack because the sucker puncher's *only* experience with fighting is fighting itself. Real fighting is all he knows, while for the karate guy, pretend fighting is all he knows. In contrast to our first example where the karate guy goes off in rage, the karate dancer may attempt or even execute some karate techniques. Only the moves won't help him much at all. In fact, his attempts at karate technique are more likely to just set him up for his assailant's perfect power shot. This is because he is not really fighting; he is *doing something about fighting.* Try to grasp what that statement means.

A Familiar Tale of a Karate Dancer

To underscore some of the points I am trying to get across regarding the delusional mind-set that afflicts so many students of karate (or any other martial art system, for that matter) until they are faced with the reality of an actual fight, I shall impart to you a tale related to me by a former bouncer and karate instructor, Mr. George Kalishevich.

Mr. Kalishevich described this little drama, which I have seen a number of variations on myself, in a letter. Having received his permission to do so, I shall relate it to you in his own words.

> I was bouncing at Bill Walker's in the Pocono Mts. resort area where I live. At about 9:30 p.m., two youngsters (I guess about 21-22 years of age) came in and sat at the bar. They were loud from the very beginning. A gentleman about 45-50 years old was at the end of the bar. He was quiet and bothering no one. One of the youngsters went over toward him and started hassling him. My fellow bouncer went over to the youngster and told him to cool it and enjoy the beer.
>
> Well, the warning was ignored not once but twice, so we escorted the youngster and his

friend, who was also starting to get cocky, out the door. About ten minutes later the older man also left.

Suddenly, a customer came running in and told us there was a big fight in the parking lot. When we got out there, one of the youngsters was flat on his ass by his car, and the other one threw a few beautifully executed roundhouse kick toward the older man's head, threw a shuto which was classical, and missed with every move right in front of the old gent.

Then the kid *simply choked up.* He saw that his karate did nothing. That's when the older man moved in with a fast left jab and right cross which put him on his back. By then, we calmed the older man down. His fury was something to see.

I can guarantee you that neither of those youngsters had *ever* been in a real fight. The older guy simply said, "Hell, I didn't want any trouble, I didn't want to fight!"

It was very obvious that he had more than his share of experience in the streets, the bars, and pool halls.

Mr. Kalishevich continued in his letter with an observation on sport karate.

Today's martial arts are too wrapped up in sport, trophies, and "champions" to be of much use on the street. They don't teach all the stuff leading up to a fight, the attitudes and mental mind-set you MUST have during a fight. The "experts" and "Masters" and "Grand Masters" who teach the bullshit taught today have never even seen, let alone been in, a real fight.

I must agree with the essence of these statements. Many of the people teaching martial arts today do not have much if any real fight experience and confuse martial arts with self-defense primarily because they don't have the background to appreciate the difference. On the other hand, there are plenty of good people out there teaching classical arts in an effective fashion. The individual instructor is always more important than the particular system being taught.

I don't take the position that it is necessary for an instructor to have a few street fights under his "belt" in order to teach effective self-defense. To the contrary, I have seen instructors who have never been in a real fight in their lives turn out some plenty tough fighters—fighters I would not want to have to face. The essential thing is that we not confuse *art* with *application*. Martial arts study itself is just that—the study of an *art*. It is not the study of applied self-defense; nor, in most cases, was it ever intended to be. (I will go into this further in a later chapter.)

A Brawl I Witnessed Involving More than a Dozen Black Belts

This tale is presented to you because it is a very real-world example of what can happen when persons skilled in classical martial arts face their first real fight.

I was a spectator at a very significant martial arts tournament. This was a full-contact, no-pads-or-gloves contest that consistently draws fighters from Europe and Asia. As guests of the sponsoring martial arts school, I and my instructors had very good, nearly ringside seats to the spectacle (made me feel like somebody).

It is significant to note that the rules of this tournament prohibit hand blows to the head or neck, but full-power kicks to the head are perfectly acceptable. The reason, of course, is that hand blows to the head are so much more effective than kicks that if they were permitted, too many people would get seriously hurt.

Also, I believe the Japanese master who sponsors the tournament (who is, incidentally, one of the best karate fighters I have ever seen, as well as a very decent, though distant, man) does not allow hands to the head to keep it a more traditional karate contest.

At one point in this tournament, a match was stopped because one fighter apparently injured a foot or toe and the referee was determining whether the fight should continue. Meanwhile, the injured fighter's manager was calling out some instructions to his fighter from ringside. He may have been saying he was going to throw in the towel, because his fighter yelled back at him some protest, obviously quite angry.

Then it happened.

Another referee, a Japanese man, began to pull the fighter's manager away from the ringside. When the Japanese referee touched the fighter's manager, the fighter exited the ring immediately and attacked the Japanese referee. It then became an instant "Katie-bar-the-door" free-for-all slugfest.

A group of perhaps six Japanese people, all in white gis and wearing black belts, rushed to the defense of the referee, who may have been their instructor. Instantly, a similar number of fighters who were part of the entourage of the contestant who started the whole thing (all dressed in black pants and black T-shirts) joined in the festivities. There were about five or six individual fights going on now.

Everybody fighting was fairly young, in good physical condition, and a black belt in one or more martial arts. Despite this (or as a result?), nobody was landing any good shots, and nobody was getting hurt. It was what my training staff refers to as "flailing" behavior (that is, people were so "pumped up" to hit somebody that they were trying to execute every technique they knew but completely ineffectually), a flurry of blows that carried no focus or power. For the most part, the blows did not connect at all or do any damage when they did. (But you know that any of these fighters would have been able to break a stack of boards with their shots in a dojo or shopping mall demonstration of karate's awesome power.)

At one point, the original fighter who left the ring returned to it to use the elevated platform to launch a running, flying sidekick to the head of a guy involved in an upper body struggle with one of his entourage. Even this blow, though it connected, only knocked the guy down for a moment. Then he sprang right back up to continue his rather ineffectual struggle with his equally ineffectual opponent.

I very clearly saw one guy in the black uniform choking a Japanese man (who was wearing a gi and black belt) with a simple front choke. The guy had both hands at the man's throat. Now, dear reader, any first-month karate student is shown how to escape this clumsy attack. I have no doubt that the Japanese man being strangled both knew and taught a number of techniques for escaping and countering it. But did I see him execute any such defensive technique? No, I did not. What I saw was the Japanese man frantically fighting at the hands at his throat (contesting the enemy's power), just as any completely untrained individual might do.

The police were not about to intervene, and the battle ended when some of the combatants in black showed the initiative and good judgment to drag their fighter out of the arena area, which put an end to this rather disgraceful spectacle. I felt bad for the karate master who sponsored the tournament. For a man of such genuine honor, it was a shameful display to have to endure.

The lesson in this incident is that the karate fighters were completely ineffectual because, although they knew techniques, they were overcome by the adrenal rush of their first actual fight. Thus, those techniques were not *accessible to* them. This is quite common, even the norm.

Not so long ago I had the fortunate opportunity to meet briefly with Stephen Hayes, who essentially introduced the art of ninjitsu to the United States. Mr. Hayes spent some time in Japan, learned to speak Japanese, and to the best of my knowledge became the first Caucasian to be admitted to the ninja ryu (school or clan), a ryu in which he has now earned senior ranking (no small accomplishment as far as your humble narrator is concerned, and one deserving of admiration and respect). As an interesting side note, Mr. Hayes has directed and served as part of the security for the Dalai Lama of Tibet.

My brief (an hour or two) training session in Mr. Hayes' dojo with some of his advanced students was followed by a short and satiric talk between the two of us about the hype and fads that the martial arts have gone through over the last 20 years.

The ability not to take oneself too seriously is to me the mark of the more advanced and enlightened individual. I found Mr. Hayes to be such an individual, and it was a real pleasure to see it. We discussed why it is that some people study martial arts and become competent fighters while most do not develop such self-defense ability. While we articulated our perceptions on this in different ways, the essence of our understanding, if I may presume to say so, seemed to be essentially the same.

Mr. Hayes made two remarks that struck me as particularly significant concerning the relationship between classical martial arts and actual combat, as well as the misunderstanding so many martial students have about the role of "technique" in a real battle.

First, he basically compared the way many people seem to think of a martial arts technique to a screwdriver that you take out of the box: you use it and it works the same way every time. He pointed to this perception as being a fundamental conceptual error because the variables present in an actual battle—even slight things such as differences in angle of attack, speed, timing, initial body position, physical setting, and so on—make every such real-world encounter a unique event. Thus, any technique has to be *applied* somewhat differently each time it is used.

I'm in full agreement with Mr. Hayes on this point. In my own books and videos, I have tried to get across this same idea, one expression of which is, "Concepts are more important than specific techniques." In fact, in actual combat, sometimes you will have to make up the technique on the spot to meet the situation at hand. This is only possible after the concepts have been internalized. A strong study of techniques can be the road to achieving this, but if you only command specific *tech-*

niques without understanding and then internalizing the *concepts* inherent in those movements, then you will be handicapped in a real fight.

The other analogy Mr. Hayes drew was that of soldiers marching on the drill field and martial arts students doing katas en masse in the dojo. While each of these activities has some value and may even be necessary, neither has anything to do with actual fighting. Nor, will either activity by itself—no matter how well it is performed or how many years it is practiced—adequately prepare someone for a real fight.

I believe that classical martial arts training is too often taught in a way that places exaggerated emphasis on form in the same way that ballet instruction does and with the same objective in mind—that is, so it *looks right* when performed. This looks-right or looks-pretty form may not always have any relevance to getting speed, power, or deception into the technique. Further, this one "true form" for executing the technique is seldom the *only* way to perform it effectively in an actual battle. Worst of all, it may be completely impractical for an actual fight in the real world. If a technique or form is not relevant or practical for a real fight, then it is a liability to try to execute it in that situation.

Most karate styles are preoccupied with doing specific techniques in very specific, prescribed ways. Stringing these specific movements into a prescribed sequence is called a *kata* or *hyung* (depending on if it's Japanese karate or Korean tae kwon do), and the whole idea is to do it exactly the same way every time.

As I see it, the only legitimate self-defense-oriented reason to emulate someone else's particular performance of a technique or series of techniques is so that you can first get a grasp of the concept upon which the technique works. In fact, this may be necessary before you can adapt the movement to your own height, size, weight, and other personal attributes. Some of this involves just the mechanics of how to do it, and emulation is an appropriate method of *initial* instruction. However, once you understand the concept upon which the technique turns, you must begin to experiment with the infinite variations in its execution such as may come up in the dynamic action of a real attack. It is unlikely that the one specific form of executing the technique learned in the kata will be the appropriate application for the specifics of an attack experienced in a real fight. Plenty of people can win kata competitions and look real sharp. But only a very few of them have any fighting ability, and fewer still any fighting experience.

This is not to say that there is no value in art. Please understand, I am referring only to preparing someone to use martial tools effectively in a real battle. That is self-defense. I am not criticizing classical martial arts themselves. After all, how can you have an art unless you maintain some conventions and formalities? Perhaps more importantly, how can any art be maintained from generation to generation unless its forms are practiced and its traditions respected? The answer is that it cannot. Thus, those who instruct and practice classical arts bear a special, necessary, and important responsibility, because without such people, these arts would soon be lost to us. There is also something to be said for art for the sake of art itself. Art shows us beauty, and, like humor, how sad our lives would be without it. Beyond even this, I have never met a really good and complete fighter who had not made a study of some classical art.

The value of classical training and, in particular, the performance of forms depends on proper attitude on the part of the practitioner. This means doing the forms with sincerity, imagining the face and attack of the assailant with fidelity. Kata should be performed as rehearsal for combat, never simply to earn a belt level or to look pretty and win some garish trophy. This would be disgraceful.

Using Techniques as Tools for Understanding Concepts

The point of all this is, if you do not have your mind right, then a knowledge of any style's techniques will be of no use in a real fight. Also, even if you are reasonably prepared for combat psychologically, if you do not understand the true role of techniques in combat, if you don't appreciate that concept is more important than technique, then you will be a mechanical robot fighter who can be easily defeated. By "robot fighter," I mean one who is incapable of adapting to unique situations, is not self-programming, and is unable to flow with the enemy.

What we are going to look at in this book demands some level of appreciation for the ideas presented in my previous work. To be more specific, you should understand that for any martial technique to work for you in an actual attack, *you must meet the following criteria first:*

1) *Your awareness level must be such that you spot the guy's opening interview,* be it verbal or nonverbal, coarse or subtle, and thus make yourself alert. You know, on some level, that the guy is thinking about the attack (at the very least) at some instant before he actually and fully executes his first attack.

2) *You must be reasonably relaxed in both body and mind,* without thought of contesting power. In short, you have your mind right and you just step up and do it.

3) *Most obviously of all, you must have practiced the techniques* with training partners until you have got the concept and can always "get" the technique (at least in the dojo-type scenarios). I think videos help a lot here, but they are of slight value if you don't have some reasonable amount of training time with a partner.

Dojos, with all their problems, are a good place to start if only because they provide people to practice with. Besides, it's the individual instructor more than even the particular art that makes a dojo what it is. A good instructor is rare and priceless.

CHAPTER TWO

Strategy, Tactics, and Technique

This chapter will further communicate the true role of physical martial technique in actual combat, the objective being to provide you with a better context in which to absorb the combat applications of any martial arts technique you might be exposed to. In addition, I want you to think about the idea that technique has to do with individual tactics, but in a real battle your overall strategy is at least as important to the outcome as any tactical application of technique.

Your tactical handling of a situation begins long before any blows are struck—even before the first woof if you are alert. Recognizing the interview and shutting it down or derailing it is the principal self-defense strategy. The things we do or say to effect this strategy are themselves techniques.

In communicating these things, I must draw not only from my own experience but from some of the knowledge and fighting experiences of my companions, the Amazing Eagle (Mike Haynack) the Mad Chinaman (Robert Stein), and others. These guys are some of my demented ex-bouncer pals and are "legendary coolers," having worked as head slammers in such ungodly establishments as the Last Resort and Duke Max's. These places make the bar in Star Wars look like the local Elk's Club. The Last Resort, however, was not located at the Moss Isley Spaceport but in a far worse hive of villainy—namely, the gambling districts of that filthiest and most utterly depraved of all these 50 states, New Jersey!

While I will draw on examples from the combat applications and philosophy of aikido, my study of aikido has been pretty brief. I do not hold myself out as being very knowledgeable of this complex and advanced art. A portion of the aikido instruction that I have received, brief though it may have been, was from a true master (and master instructor), namely, Shihan Fumio Toyoda-San of the Aikido Association of America in Chicago. The bulk of my aikido instruction has been from Mike Haynack and the Mad Chinaman. Both Mike and the Chinaman slam with beauty, have combat experience, and understand the expression "harmony or else." Both practice Toyoda-San's, Chicago-style aikido.

Chicago-style aikido is the true aikido that rips the dogs out of the ground and sends them hurling through space or, alternatively, crunches them "in place," therefore restoring harmony to the universe. If you want to see this kind of aikido, go to Chicago and see the master at work in his dojo on West Belmont Avenue. Take your shoes off and bow when you enter the dojo, and be polite (that's a tip, people).

Previously, I said that a sense of humor, even self-parody, is a mark of the more enlightened individual. Shihan Toyoda-San certainly has these qualities since he awarded me my fukushidoin (assistant instructor) certification in aikido because, as he put it, "... strong a spirit you are a having."

Simultaneously with presenting this award, he

leaned over and spoke in my ear the caution, "But, you wanna be teaching any aikido, you better coming to see me first." What a character! His technique has to be experienced to be believed. Toyoda-San is one of a handful of true living masters that I have had the good fortune to have been slammed by. (Later in this book we will look at what makes a "master," why there are so few of them, and why it can be counterproductive to try to emulate too precisely the way of a master in your own martial study.)

Once again, you are cautioned that I am no instructor of aikido. Having given you these warnings, I will now presume to tell you that many of the things I did in the bar—having never really even seen aikido before—I later discovered were formalized as "arts" in aikido. They are called arts, I believe, because the emphasis is on the concept rather than on any specific application of the concept as may be reflected in a particular technique. Hence, in aikido, there are infinite variations on a given technique like ikkyo. They may look like very different techniques; still, they are all called ikkyo because they are all based on the ikkyo concept.

Aikido in general is more concept- and less technique-oriented than other martial arts. This makes it somewhat more advanced in its approach. Because of that advancement, this art may be starting too far down the line for many people to grasp its combat relevance. But to be a well-rounded fighter you need exposure to more than one or two martial systems. This is because the strategic approaches of different martial arts can be quite different. If you study only a single art, you are limiting yourself to that art's particular strategic approach.

For example, the basic strategic approach of karate is to defeat the enemy with powerful striking techniques to the most vulnerable areas and nerve centers of the enemy's body. In contrast, the basic strategic approach in aikido is to slip or blend with the attack so as to be able to redirect it and thus achieve the beauty slam (throw). In judo the strategy is also based on breaking the enemy's balance, but this is accomplished by the "aikido-like blending" only at its highest levels of practice. Otherwise, the judo strategy is to enter and knock the enemy's balance from him by striking with the hip to his pelvis so that his weight is relieved from his feet, and then using the hip as a fulcrum for the leverage throw. Once the enemy's feet leave the ground, he becomes weightless and thus the severity of the fall can be controlled to achieve the desired effect (sport or bone-cracking slam). The Brazilian jujutsu strategy is to close on the enemy and grapple to deny him the opportunity to strike powerfully and then take him to the ground where his striking technique is of little value to him. On the ground he is quite vulnerable to the choke or joint lock. This strategy forces the enemy to fight on the ground, which he is unfamiliar with and the Brazilian jujutsu man is quite accomplished at.

If you begin to think more in terms of the concepts on which a technique turns (rather than the specific techniques themselves), then it will be easier for you to learn new approaches, new arts, and the new strategic approaches that manifest themselves in those arts' techniques. So when examining a new martial art, try to first identify the overall strategy of the art rather than just its particular techniques.

It is sometimes necessary in our training to change our conceptual, mental approach to dealing with an attack in order to learn the techniques and the strategic emphasis of a new and unfamiliar martial system. An example is found in teaching hard-style karate people some aikido. Because the hard-style karate concept is grounded mostly in power striking from a solid foundation, it is more difficult for karate people (at first, anyway) to learn to flow and spin and "mirror an attack." But it is just these concepts that provide the opportunity for the righteous aikido-style slam. And what bone-splintering beauty such a slam can truly be.

SOMETIMES YOU NEED TO BLAST, SOMETIMES YOU NEED TO SLAM

Sometimes you need to blast with a power strike, but

there are also times when its better to slip the bastard's blow and slam the behemoth into a solid object. Allow me to digress into a personal example.

Fights can start over the stupidest shit. In fact, people are killed over the stupidest shit. Fortunately, that didn't happen in the tale I shall now relate. I was in a very crowded bar in New Mexico. (This was the same town I would work in as a bouncer.) The bar was packed three or four deep, and I really wasn't enjoying the atmosphere of this place at all. Too crowded, too much noise, and too many cowboys trying to play hard guy. But, since I had driven all the way into town to have a beer, it was in my mind to do just that and then go home.

I don't wait in line very well so it was an exercise in self discipline for me to wait for the barkeep to serve those in front of me before I could get that beer. But I could see that he was moving as fast as he could back there. Finally, when my beer was set down in front of me, I was definitely ready for it. But a second after it hit the bar, a unseen person behind me reached past me to snatch my beer for himself. As I intercepted his hand reaching for my beer, I felt his arm begin its turn for the attack. (All this stuff happened in about one-thirtieth of a second.) Feeling his hostile action (in progress), I reflexively slipped to his elbow and threw him . . . and he went, too.

Once again, there are some techniques that don't look like much in the dojo, but when a person gives you a real attack you get that real juice (inertia, movement) to work with. These are the conditions where sometimes a classical technique can work like magic—particularly when it's the first physical contact in the conflict.

Ordinarily my move would not have thrown a person, particularly a guy this big. But, because in that next instant he turned just right and so decisively and powerfully, and because my step was good, his feet left the ground and he landed flat on his ass. At that point I saw that the guy I was having this altercation with for the first time. This guy could have been a stand-in for Arnold

Schwarzenegger body-wise, and I was not interested in fighting him if I didn't have to.

I raised both my hands, empty palms toward him in a gesture of "there is no need to fight over this" and I stepped back a little. It was possible for me to step back now because a vacuum had just occurred in the dense crowd around us. I knew this guy might go for it now because there was such an obvious audience that he might feel he had to "redeem" himself. He stepped in immediately and threw a right hook to my head. I was perceptually ready for this blow, and I was looking right at him; thus, I was able to respond. I closed inside his range before his shot landed, and his arm impacted on the back of my shoulder.

From this impact it was clear to me that this guy was so big I could not afford to take even one of his shots, but after I'd hit him about four times in his gut (karate reverse-punch style) in about one and a half seconds, I knew something else . . . namely, that my hands hurt because his gut was so hard.

When he threw his next shot I ducked under it and slid behind and past him. I saw it in his face for a moment, the recognition that he might be dealing with a trained fighter. But sadly, I definitely did not see in that face any concern over this discovery.

Since I knew I probably couldn't hurt this guy by striking him, I immediately gave up any such idea and my movements became directed not toward affording the opportunity for a counterstrike, but only toward avoiding his strike and any upper body struggle where I would be overpowered.

But this guy was pumped and swinging fast. He moved pretty damn good, especially for such a big, muscular guy (adrenaline does this), and though I avoided taking his shots, he had me inside again and was grabbing my left arm to hold me for his next shot.

We were now in that upper body struggle that I had hoped to avoid. When I felt him grab my left arm I stepped past again for a usoto gari throw. It failed at first, but from previous experience and training I knew just to lean into it with my full body weight and whack his leg again with everything I had. I did, and he went down all at once and pretty hard.

In retrospect, always 20-20, it could have been a mistake for me to allow him to get back up. But I didn't think I had a shot powerful enough to finish him, so I was still thinking in terms of keeping some distance and letting him hurl himself at me so I could sail him into something.

Nowadays, I know a better solution to this problem, which is the "knee strike to the head" on a enemy who is rising from the ground; back then I didn't. If I had trained on that technique before this incident, I believe I would have been able to knock him out with it. He definitely made the technique "available" to me when he was getting up.

But, "all's well that ends well," and when he did get back up he was a shade slower than before. He had been hit hard enough to daze him a little, but his rage was only slightly abated if at all. He then overextended in his blood lust to get me. His attack was a rhino that might have included an overhand right, but he never got the shot off because I spun him into the bar using a variation of the old "one up, one down" as the Eagle refers to it.

His forehead and some of his face hit the bar edge first and that did the trick. He was semiconscious (though he was getting up) when suddenly, two even bigger guys showed up who were the bouncers in this place.

As the previous tale illustrates, sometimes you have to be able to change strategies in the middle of a fight. You can't begin to do this if you choke (or are in a blind rage). Once you get past the choke reaction, techniques that are not otherwise possible become possible. Once you get past the blind rage stage, it becomes possible to make transitions in your fighting strategy should the combat demand same.

The real trick in doing this is to first develop some ability to do either (i.e., blast or slam, strike or throw), and then to be able to make the instantaneous transitions from one mind-set to the other (under adrenal fight

TWO VERSIONS OF A RIGHTEOUS SLAM JOB

There are many kinds of beauty. The two throws shown here are "combat" versions of the ones I used most frequently in my bouncer work. On pavement, being thrown like this could be fatal because the back of the person's head will often impact first. With skill one can learn to control the severity of this fall and avoid this. But here the technique is shown in its full combat style.

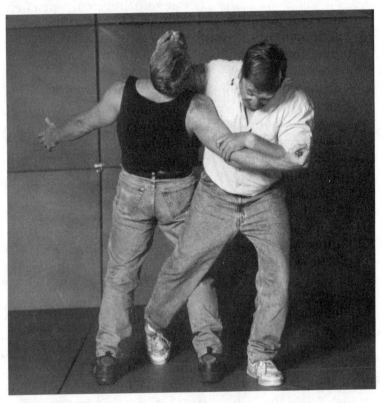

Note that my right hand has slapped down over his face (perhaps breaking his nose) and pushed his head back so that he is looking straight up. My left hand has captured his elbow, pulling it behind him as I step past him. Observe that my left foot is actually behind his right foot when my right leg sweeps out his left leg. This is a combat version of the classic judo throw usoto gari. Notice my projection of intent as I look down and past him to the spot where he is about to be slammed. This is the same concept as follow-through in a golf swing. It helps ensure a smooth and complete movement.

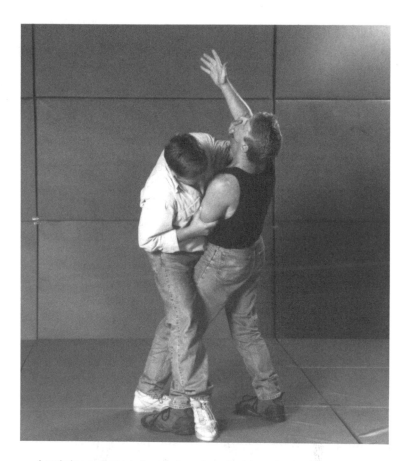

A variation on the technique that employs all of the same concepts. Here I may have ducked or preempted a shot from his right hand as I drop my head out of the path of the blow and enter on the enemy. My left hand has struck him under the jaw with a rising heel of palm strike. This knocks his head back so that he is again looking almost straight up. But my right leg has hooked behind his left leg and thus he cannot stay on his feet. In this frame, his right hand has flown up as his balance is broken, and he will fall straight back. This technique is easier to control in terms of how severely the person hits the asphalt or floor.

stress) as the circumstances of the combat may require. This is difficult but far from impossible and depends primarily on having been previously trained realistically and under adrenal stress conditions.

YOUR PHYSICAL RESPONSES MUST BE PROGRAMMED INTO YOUR MUSCULAR MEMORY

Now, some people reading this, particularly if they have been in a few street scraps, might say, "What are you talking about? In a fight you just gotta go for it, 'cause once it's on, it's fucking on, and you better go after the bastard with everything you have. There's no time to 'think' about strategy in a real fight—shit, a real fight only lasts a few seconds anyway!"

In fact, this was part of what I tried to get across in my first book. Further, I will acknowledge that the above mind-set is a good one to have for battle. Indeed, it may be the best attitude toward a fight that most people can achieve. But this mind-set is somewhat kindred to the blind rage that I talked about in the previous chapter. As such, it limits the use of higher brain functions that are capable of strategically adapting despite the confusion of an adrenal episode (such as a fight). In military parlance, this adrenal-based confusion is often referred to as the "fog of battle."

However, if one is accustomed to some level of adrenal stress (having experienced it before), it certainly is possible to make these mental transitions during combat. This transition must first occur in the combat mind-set itself before it can express itself in a change in physical technique or strategy.

It is exactly because there really is no time to think about anything in a real fight that your body and muscular memory must do most of this transitional work for you—and do it under the adrenal stress of battle. Unfortunately, it is precisely because most people have a lack of experience with real fighting and the adrenal reaction that accompanies it that they encounter their biggest problems in an actual fight.

The obvious solution is to devise a method of training that gives these people the adrenal stress experience and then allows them to execute full-force techniques while under such adrenalization. This is the mechanism by which muscular memory is formed. That is exactly what we do in our combat applications method of scenario training in Colorado. I submit that the results achieved by this method are testament to the fact that it is the adrenal stress effects that cause people their real problems in a fight rather than their limited or imperfect knowledge of technique. Further, once people develop some level of adrenal conditioning, they are much better able to absorb and retain physical technique, and then it becomes the adrenal response itself that "cues up" this ability to execute technique properly and with power.

But an exposition of the training method we employ at our Colorado facility and the weekend programs is the subject of the next chapter. First, let's consider the four basic strategic approaches to combat.

THE "BIG FOUR" ELEMENTS OF STRATEGY IN PERSONAL COMBAT

A strategy is an overall approach to a problem. Tactics are the specific things we do to effect our strategy. As this applies to combat, strategy has to do with overall concepts, while tactics are specific techniques.

For example, there are many techniques for sweeping out an enemy's leg so that he falls down hard. The concept upon which these techniques turn (that is, the strategy) is simply to break the opponent's balance. No sweeping technique will ever drop a man if you do not first break his balance. Conversely, you can execute almost any technique successfully once you do break an opponent's balance.

The significance of this is that once you truly understand the concept of breaking someone's balance, you will discover an infinite variety of techniques with which to achieve this. More importantly, you will be moving toward that goal of being able to discover or invent specific techniques during the battle itself as are required and as your enemy makes them available. This is sometimes referred to as "flow."

The Big Four elements of combat strategy that we will look at are as follows:

1) Breaking the enemy's balance
2) Blending with and redirecting the enemy's attack
3) Trapping and immobilizing the enemy's defense
4) Preempting the enemy's attack
   (Stopping the enemy's mind)

Note that things like using the environment as a weapon may be seen more as techniques than strategies because to do them we first must have effected one of these Big Four general strategies. For example, strategies #1 and #2 most often precede the "use of environment as a weapon" techniques.

Even as I write these strategic elements down, salty and nostalgic tears nearly come to my eyes as I recall their splendor as expressed by my having applied them successfully in a particular past combat. I guess that's a sure sign that I'm getting old. Perhaps I should indulge myself and share one of those fond memories with you.

A Primitive but Effective Application
of Breaking the Enemy's Balance

Sometimes in the bar work (this was long before the legal liability issue got out of hand), situations would arise where patrons were "cut off" but flatly refused to leave and loudly demanded to be served.

These people were not always drunk either, or at least many times they would not appear to be drunk by most people's standards. Many times, the bartender simply cut them off because they were being obnoxious and were verbally molesting other patrons. This made them very bad for the barkeep's business, since he relied heavily on tips from happy customers. With these loud "problem patrons," the objective was to see to it that they did not become regulars, since their behavior was unwanted. We therefore needed to make them feel unwanted in our establishment.

This one guy was just such an individual, and he was telling me, as the Eagle might put it, that (1) he had money, (2) he was going to be served another drink, and (3) there was nothing I could do about it. He was quite a large person—well over six foot, maybe 245 pounds; about 35 to 37 years old; and he looked thick and powerful. I was about 27 at the time, standing a whopping 5-foot-9-1/2 inches tall, and weighing about 190 pounds.

I observed that the front two legs of his stool, the ones closest to the bar, would raise from the floor occasionally as he moved and rocked back a bit in his seat while one or both of his hands were on the bar. The dude was making it very easy for me to apply the "breaking the enemy's balance" element of combat strategy. So rather than trying to wrench this behemoth out of his stool (contesting the enemy's power), that is exactly what I did by hooking my foot on the leg of his stool. Then, while talking to him calmly, and while he began to amp up his woofing, I suddenly whipped out the stool from under him with my foot just as his weight shifted. He naturally fell over backward and hit the floor (use of environment as a weapon). It was then a fairly simple matter to apply the ubiquitous arm bar on him and roll him over on his belly before he was able to get up from the floor (continuous attack).

The combination of the arm bar and my body weight pressing down on him while he was belly down made it quite difficult for him to get up and do anything, though his initial efforts toward that end were quite vigorous and sincere. I also chose this position for him in case he turned out to be a "berzerker." In such a case I could go directly to the rear choke, and once I got that on him his size, power, and berzerker attitude would be of no use to him at all. The choke would have him unconscious in a matter of 10 seconds or less.

Whipping out the stool from under him can be seen

as preempting the enemy's attack. The turnover and then the arm bar are very low-level examples of trapping the enemy's defense. The guy swore and screamed out all the things he was going to do to me when he got up, so I just let him struggle himself out to near exhaustion. I needed to use very little effort, mostly just my body weight to keep him down.

Not a real exciting story, I know. The thing that makes it stick in my mind, I guess, is how effortless it all was. The guy was really big, but I never gave him a chance to use his power. Had it gone to a fist fight, I could have had some real problems with a guy that big. Because I understood the concept of breaking the enemy's balance and had some experience in doing so, I acted with confidence and just whomped the stool out from under him, sending him crashing to the floor. This is an example of proper mind, the use of an appropriate strategy for the situation, and only a little bit of luck.

Having taken the initiative with the stool move, I controlled every event that followed in the sequence, and therefore I did not have to depend on being faster than my enemy. He was preempted from responding with any attack at all. There was therefore no need for me to hurry or be anxious (in mind or body) to get things done, because I knew I had him the minute I saw him rock the legs of the stool back. All of this is part of the same whole and was made not only possible but nearly effortless because of an appreciation of the concept of breaking the enemy's balance combined with a relaxed and confident mind.

Any physical technique, or sequence of techniques, that is useful and practical in real fighting will contain all of the Big Four elements of strategy when employed in any personal combat. However, in general, one of the four—breaking the enemy's balance, blending and redirecting the enemy's attack, trapping, or preemption—will dominate the tactical sequence.

The dominant element of the tactical sequence we will examine next is preemption. I have chosen it for sticky, sentimental reasons.

The "Come See the Stars" Technique

Okay! Relax your mind and give this your full attention. The technique I'm going to describe to you now is a real treasure; what's more, you can learn to do it fairly quickly by working with a training partner. Once reasonably mastered, this technique sequence will allow you to whack almost anybody alive (whose behavior makes the technique available) right smack in the nose with plenty of juice before he even realizes it's happened, much less can do anything to stop it.

Sound too good to be true? Maybe like those "Deadly Monkey Hands of Steel" I talked about in the first paragraph of this book? Glad you think so—shows good judgment and a healthy skepticism on your part . . . makes me think I'm getting through sometimes.

Only this time, there really are some "Deadly Monkey Hands of Steel!" I could call this technique that or anything else. The only thing that can really keep you from pulling it off effectively in a real confrontation is either 1) you choke or 2) your enemy does not make the technique available.

I've selected the "come see the stars" technique partly for reasons of nostalgia. However, it does reflect all of the Big Four elements of combat strategy and serves particularly well as a means to communicate the spirit of the preemption element. You will see why as we progress.

The Situation Where the Technique Comes Up

This technique becomes available when a "hot" interviewer reaches out for you when you are both facing each other and are fairly close together. This situation will occur very often when an interviewer either 1) steps right up to you and points his finger in your face, generally while making some verbal threats, or 2) actually reaches out to grab hold of you. (This grab is often used to hold the victim for the punch.)

In the latter case, we assume your awareness level has been sufficient to have recognized this hot stage of the interview. You know the interviewer's attack is imminent (as Master Toyoda might say, "He is a grabbing for you, for

HOW THE MOST COMMON "PUNCH-OUT" OCCURS

Perhaps the original beef is over a fender-bender-type auto accident or such. It could be any number of things, but here is the basic modus operandi of many a punch-out, and it is simple in the extreme.

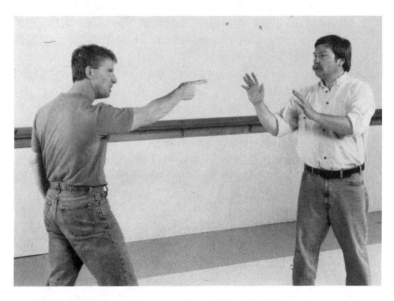

We hear the woof, as in, "You stupid son of a bitch!" We see the pointing gesture directed toward us and the anger and hatred in the guy's face. The thing to understand is that the "fight" has actually already begun at this point.

As quick and "red hot" as it is, this is still an interview. The failure to defend was primarily a failure to recognize the "hot interview." Even if the victim simply dropped his head so that he took the impact of the fist on the hard part of his skull, this closed fist blow could likely break the assailant's hand on impact. I have seen broken hands happen like that more than once, and it most often takes the fight right out of the sucker puncher.

A better way to handle this situation would be by pre-emption. Once you see he is going to attack, beat him to the punch and forestall his attack with one of your own. This demands self-confidence, both in your judgment that preemption is necessary and in your ability to drop your assailant.

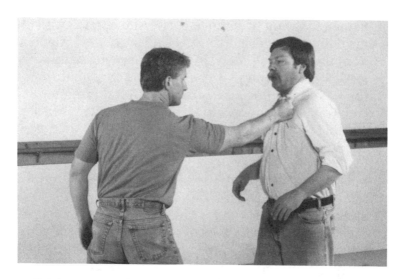

But since most people are not accustomed to this type of stand-up agression, they hesitate because they are essentially in denial of the fact that it is really happening. Their mind is divided because a portion is saying, "This can't really be happening; he must be crazy." Then immediately comes the grab, physical contact that follows the invasive pointing gesture. The attack is now on its way.

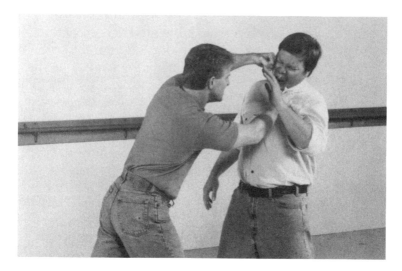

"ZANGO!" The assailant has stabilized the target with his grab of the victim's clothing and now throws the overhead punch to the head. The assailant will then immediately continue with follow-up shots and put the victim away, never giving him a chance to defend himself or "come back" (continuous attack).

to punching you"). In the first case, the interview is still at the pointing stage, but you "feel" that a second later it will be at the grabbing stage. In either case, you have already made the decision that you are going to drop this guy to the pavement because in your rational judgment (not macho-man-madness thinking and not out of fear), you feel that this is your best (safest) self-defense strategy.

An extreme example of such a situation (one of many) would be when there are two guys confronting you and one is clearly the "mouth." He is the guy who will conduct the interview and then initiate the attack. There is also no way to just run for it with any decent expectation of escaping these assailants, and you have foolishly found yourself unarmed. Your awareness level is sufficiently developed for you to perceive that the mouth's companion (a "pilot fish") will wait for the leader to attack first before he joins in on the assault and tries to stomp on you. You see that this is where it's going if you don't handle it correctly by shutting down the interview. You will shut down the interview . . . by dropping the interviewer.

As I've said, avoidance is your best strategy. Preemption can be seen as an advanced and proactive form of avoidance. You will avoid having to fight both guys (and likely being beat up real bad or worse) by taking out the first guy (the mouth) first and thus hopefully avoiding the fight altogether—or at least avoiding having to fight two guys all at once (since the mouth should already be down). You will not wait around for the leader to be ready to get things rolling with his own attack.

If things work well, once the other guy sees the leader hit the floor and he feels you project heavily on him (sometimes called extending your ki power), he will hesitate and likely not attack immediately. This may allow you to escape.

The whole deal—once you drop the guy having executed your "come see the stars" technique—should take maybe one and a half or two seconds before you are headed down the street, out the door, or into your car as the case may be.

You should not mistake this to mean that only a "real fast guy" can get away with this. You may recall the three components of speed, as discussed in my first book. The first is perception. You must first percieve that your enemy is preparing an attack by recognizing his body carriage, his walk, his facial expression, and so on as hostile even before he gets to the pointing gesture part of the interview. The second component is the selection of a response. Your response to the pointing woofer should have been decided and practiced long before you ran into this particular woofer. So there is no delay in selecting your response. The final component is the velocity with which you execute the chosen response. Since the "come see the stars" technique does not require us to tense either our muscles or our mind, this final component of speed, execution of the technique itself, can be very fast.

Most people can execute this technique before their enemy can do anything to stop or block it . . . if they simply relax their minds, which relaxes their muscles, and then they just step up and do it. Remember, the primary point of explaining this technique is to illuminate the concept of preemption. In a preemptive move you seize the initiative by acting first. This forces your enemy to try to react in time to defeat your movement. Action is always faster than reaction. This reality is at the core of all preemptive attacks.

Now let's look at the mechanics of the technique. Study the photos on pages 44-45 and appreciate the mechanics of the movement, simple as it is. Practice both sides (right and left) with your training partner once you've got your strong side down well.

Understand that this level of violence is only warranted because I know exactly what the assailant is going to do before he completes his action. He intends to freeze me in place with the woof so he can grab my shirt collar and punch me out. His woof and invasive pointing gesture are his preparation for this attack, even though they only take a second or two before he actually throws the punch. The best time to attack is on the enemy's preparation to attack.

THE "COME SEE THE STARS" TECHNIQUE

This technique is really quite simple, as any technique must be if it is to be useful in an actual situation. It is the spirit of preemption and *timing* that make this technique work in a real confrontation. The entire sequence is continuous but is broken down into three parts below to show the mechanics . . . and it all takes less than one second to execute. This technique is also useful against the attempted grab.

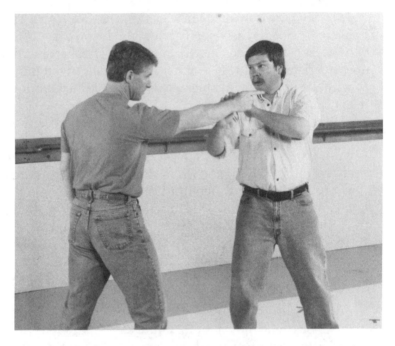

The instant I see the pointing gesture and the woof and the enemy closing on me, I know the attack is in progress. Without hesitation I step directly into the enemy. My right hand crosses my own centerline and "pats" his arm (my hand brushes across the arm, drawing it slightly toward me) as I step into the pointing woofer.

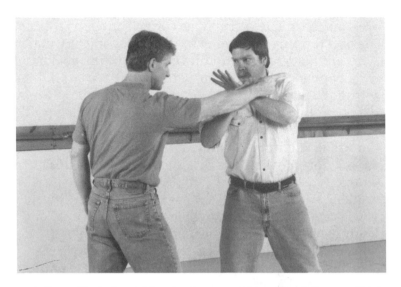

In the next instant my left hand replaces my right on his pointing arm. This is not a push and certainly not a grab, but only a light tap or pat.

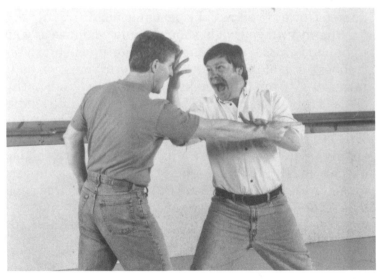

As my left replaces my right hand, my right hand comes off his arm and it flops into the enemy's face, striking and breaking the nose. While I have had this strike achieve the knockout directly, it should be thought of as a set-up shot and must be followed up with continuous attack (shutos to the carotid artery after peeling the head back, a throw like usoto gari.)

This technique, when done correctly, is also an example of "stopping the enemy's mind." You might wonder, why not just step in and blast him with the backhand strike and skip all the arm-patting stuff? Well, if done without any hesitation, that might work, too. But the enemy's mind is often engaged by the unexpected tactile sensation of this double tap on his arm, and that sets up the strike and draws him into it (it also indexes your own strike). Some martial arts disciplines might see this as an example of "tuite," or nerve activation by a triad sequence (three strikes, the first two sensitizing the nervous system for the third, which is the knockout). I don't know about all that. Maybe there is something to it, but I do know that nothing works every time in a real battle.

When the guy's left hand is extended far enough toward you that he is reaching out and is just about to make contact with you, you pivot in, just like in the inside crane technique (from *Bouncer's Guide to Barroom Brawling*). Sometimes this means you begin to step in as he steps toward you with his reaching hand.

Simply turn your right shoulder into your man as your right hand crosses over your own centerline to brush the grabber's arm along its natural arc, while your own body turns away from the attacker's anticipated grab point. (This is called "mirroring," particularly in aikido study.) Then your left hand replaces your right on the guy's arm. This is a gentle but instantaneous exchange. Your left is simply "stuck" on the guy's arm, holding it down and out of the way. But this is not truly a grab, since your arm muscles are not fully tensed. With your now free right hand, you flow into a backhand strike to your enemy's nose, which comes directly along his centerline. This blow might be called the "vertical backhand slap."

The Vertical Backhand Slap

Don't be misled by the "slap" terminology. The few times I've done this technique for real, the guys were knocked senseless, and if they did not drop to the pavement right there, it was a simple matter to follow up with knockout shots since they were momentarily helpless.

You do not waste any time or motion by turning over the hand for the heel-of-palm blow. Instead, the idea of economy of movement has led you to explore simply whacking the dude in the nose with the back of your hand—that is, instantly after the right hand comes off the arm after brushing it past.

Practice on an air shield. The blow should snap back as fast as it goes out. The hand is never tensed into a fist but remains completely relaxed until just before impact. After impact, it relaxes and snaps back, like a bullwhip.

You must use tai sabaki movement, that is, proper body weight shift so the blow, though struck very quickly with the hand, carries your full body weight.

Use your breath and voice to shout as you enter into the movement. This tends to surprise and confuse the enemy and make him more likely to tense at the critical instant.

You will likely be surprised at how easy it is to break a 12 x 12 x 1-inch pine board with this backslap blow without hurting your hand. If you can break two such boards with this technique, then you have got a shot that will knock out a good number of people. Practice on foam pads and air shields first.

Bouncer's Guide covered this idea of acceleration-based blows. It's essential for you to appreciate that concept in order to achieve power in this type of shot, the backfist, or any other acceleration-type blow. But I must assume you have some appreciation for these ideas and move ahead.

Seeing and Appreciating the Big Picture

If you have studied the photographs or the videos and worked out with a partner who plays the role of the interviewer by pointing his finger, moving close and woofing on you, then you might start thinking "Damn, it seems impossible that anybody could block this." Well, guess what? Basically, you are right. But let's examine why this is so and, more importantly, what implications this has in terms of strategy and technique and proper combat mind-set.

First, consider that the reason you can get the back-hand strike to the enemy's face before he can do anything to block it is that he has already made a critical tactical error, which you are immediately prepared (psychologically and physically) to exploit.

The error he has made is to close distance on you, moving into your range without an effective attack of his own. The pointing finger is not truly an attack. It is an intelligence-gathering probe that is also meant to intimidate you and make you tense up (not being relaxed), maybe even freeze up. When the interviewer sees this fear on your face, he will throw his shot because he knows it's safe to do so.

This can all happen at the velocity of a simple "grab and punch," though. This is why I simply do not allow people to put hands on me in any sort of manhandling fashion. If they do this, the fight is on, which means they will find themselves hurt and on the ground in the next instant. If you must fight, this is a good way to start out the battle.

The Aggressor Has a
Preconception about How You Will Behave

Have you ever seen a bully or interviewer actually poke his finger into somebody's chest two or even three times, actually pushing the guy back before throwing a right hand to his head? Maybe you have. Perhaps it was way back when, like on the playground as a child. Guess what? Bully types never really grow up. But, they often do grow larger, more dangerous, and more vicious.

Therefore, I'm saying that the guy pointing his finger at you has a given mind-set (that of the bully). This means he has a set of expectations concerning what's going to happen next, which you can often exploit.

Also note that though he may go off (throw a punch) at any instant, at the precise instant he points his finger at you he is not prepared to attack (otherwise, he would have done so). Further, his set of expectations about what is going to happen next does not include your preemption with the "come see the stars" technique. This is all part of why he has made the technique available to you.

When Has the Die Been Cast?

Now, think about this very significant question: at what point is the finger-pointing bully doomed to eat your backhand shot? The simple answer is, the instant you perceive that he is about to close the distance and make the "offering" of the finger—assuming you have made up your mind to drop him. This also assumes, of course, that you are psychologically prepared to execute the "come see the stars" technique the instant your enemy makes it available.

Again, this is why awareness and mental preparedness are everything in real-world self-defense situations. For a skilled and experienced fighter, this can mean that the finger-pointer is doomed some time before he makes any apparent move to even take those first few steps to close the distance, much less begins to raise his hand to point the finger.

This is part of what Musashi meant when he wrote, "The combat is decided before first swords are crossed." If you ponder this long enough you will see that for any particular technique (once some reasonable level of mastery has been achieved), there is a point where if the enemy assumes a given position, then he makes the technique available, and nothing can prevent its successful application—except the person executing it.

One reason I bring this up is to highlight yet another aspect of the fact that your mental attitude will be the central determinant of the outcome of a fight. If you can relax your mind when a person is trying to intimidate you (very often a precursor to a physical attack), your vision will be unrestricted; you will see everything he is doing. More importantly, you will see what he is about to do, that is, what he is working himself up to do. This allows you to anticipate his making available a given technique, and then you are right there when he does.

When you are studying a martial arts technique, make

an effort to determine what actions on the part of the assailant would make the given technique available to you. Then work backward from there and imagine the actions or behavior on the part of the hot interviewer that might likely precede those behaviors. Sometimes these mind's-eye visualization exercises may demonstrate to you that a given martial technique has virtually no application at all to a real fight because the antecedent on the part of the assailant that would make it available is not ever likely to occur.

On the other hand, if the dojo attack is an imaginary sword represented by the training partner's hand chopping straight down at your head, this does not mean the technique is automatically irrelevant to combat. Observe and appreciate the angle of attack and the precursing body cues the training partner gives to execute it. Then imagine, might someone swing a baseball bat, or tire iron, or beer bottle at you like that? How, then, would the technique need to be modified to deal with same?

When you receive instruction in any new martial arts technique, think about when the die has been cast for its effective application. This is another way of perceiving the idea of when the application of the technique becomes available.

You Cannot Execute a Technique
Successfully before the Enemy Makes it Available

Appreciate that you cannot really "force" a technique on the situation in real combat. This is a common error or fault of many an otherwise technically proficient martial artist. He tries to force his favorite technique on the combat—the one he is confident with, the one he practices in the dojo all the time. But if his enemy has not made the technique available by some action of his own, the favorite technique fails. This can have a profoundly negative effect on the martial artist's spirit and thus on his fighting attitude.

Recall Mr. Kalishnivik's tale of the old guy fighting the two karate dancers in the parking lot. The kid choked after his beautiful roundhouse to the head had no effect. The failure of a favorite technique alone decided the outcome of the battle, particularly when this failure made available to his enemy a simple and direct counterattack.

Now, think what this really means regarding the strategic use of preemption. Even perfect preemption requires some action on the part of the aggressor first that makes it possible. At the very least, and at its most subtle, this action is the aggressor's earliest expression of the interview—perhaps even his first "pose" to prepare for the opening of his interview.

Now consider this: what kind of person is it that will make the "come see the stars" technique available? Clearly, it is an aggressive person who is initiating a chain of events whereby his objective is to punch somebody out, that is, to do aggressive and unprovoked violence to somebody.

But first, he has to make sure that the punch-out prospect is safe, that is, that there isn't any significant probability of his getting hurt by fucking with the wrong guy. On some level of his mind, he has this fear. This is what is behind his conducting the interview (finger-pointing and woofing) before he does attack.

I feel that I would never be blasted by the "come see the stars" technique in the context of the situation I have described with the finger-pointing bully. Why? Is this simple arrogance on my part—a quality which I clearly have in abundance? I like to think not. The reason I don't think I'd be blasted by this move is because I would never make the technique available. In other words, I'd never treat anyone like that. I would not bully someone with a pointing-finger-type interview. If I thought I had to drop them to defend myself, I'd just do that (or try to). Further, if I did do some bullying stunt like that because I was drunk or lost control of myself in a moment of rage or whatnot, then, not only could I be dropped by this technique, I'd deserve to be dropped by it as well. My actual fighting experience has demonstrated to me the reality of this particular weakness of the bully's modus operandi.

My personal self-defense style has motivated me to ana-
lyze and exploit that weakness (as well as to appreciate
the bully's potential to inflict injury or death).

Consider the words of O'Sensei, Morihei Ueshiba, the
founder of the art of aikido:

> *Winning means winning over the discord in yourself.*
> *Those who have a warped mind, a mind of discord,*
> *have been defeated from the beginning.*

A Closing Thought on the
"Come See the Stars" Technique

If you ever have to use this move, keep in mind that
just because you might break the guy's nose right off the
bat, this does not mean he won't then grab onto you, twist
you down to the ground, and beat the bloody shit out of
you. This preemptive strike in some situations must be
followed up with continuous attack, culminating in some
type of takedown or throw or clavicle busting, etc.

Some people I have had to hit just mentally collapsed
and, holding their bloody nose, started whining something like, "You broke my fucking nose! You broke my
fucking nose!" These types suddenly forget all about playing "tough guy" and became totally preoccupied with
their own injury and pain. However, do not count on it!

Other people just go ape shit and get that heavy
adrenaline boost, then just go off in a rage to kill you.
These type of berzerkers are not so easily dealt with by
striking-type techniques unless you have a good stick. It's
often best to stay away from them so they can burn themselves out. Berzerkers do make themselves somewhat
more vulnerable to the "use of the environment as a
weapon" techniques once you have succeeded in applying a "breaking the opponent's balance" technique.

A common example is side-stepping a "rhino" attack,
then pushing the guy's head down and running him head
first into the bar, a post, or a parked car. (We will be con-
sidering all this beauty and, specifically, a training
method that helps people achieve same later.)

Don't Be the Prisoner of Your
Own Macho Madness Thinking

Now, for you people who have read my first book (and God bless you) and are maybe thinking, "Hmm, this dude's getting soft in his old age—too much time spent pounding computer keys on the word processor and too long ago since he was pounding on hard heads in the barroom," please allow me to respond.

First, it is true that it has been more than a few years since I had to actually slam anybody's head into the bar edge. In fact, it's been a while since I have had to do any real street fighting at all. But I sincerely believe this is primarily the result of my overcoming testosterone poisoning (technical term for "machismo madness") and the success of my awareness and avoidance strategy. If you are smart, it won't take you 20 years of brawling, busted bones, severe legal problems, etc., to appreciate and arrive at this attitude.

Furthermore, though it's been some years since I was a head cracker in the bars, what has really changed there? How have people really changed? If a samurai who lived centuries ago makes the same observations about the reality of fighting as I and my companions have made in 20th-century America, then it's clear that these things represent truths that are timeless and transcultural.

When I offer you O'Sensei's quote concerning the idea that those with a warped mind have lost already, I am trying to get the idea across that anyone who interviews you before the attack (and most will) does so because he is unsure of victory. He is not as totally confident as he tries to appear. He fears potential defeat.

All that is demanded for you to defeat most such individuals is your simply being aware that you are being interviewed (as early as possible) and then maintaining a relaxed mind. Then (most often) either he will decide not to press his luck and will move on to a more passive game, or, if he does decide to go for you, you are already perceptually ready for it, you see it coming, and you are able to deal with it. Don't hesitate!

The fact is, there have been more than a few occasions when people have pointed their fingers toward my face and barked out some threats in the last year or two. Because I knew on a very deep level that at any time I decided to do so, I could render these guys unconscious on the pavement, I felt no real fear and thus no real anxiousness to do so. I'll go a step further with this line of thought. Having had to drop more than a few people in such circumstances, I can say that I have only rarely experienced any real satisfaction in doing so. Generally, it's all pretty ugly and unpleasant, apart even from the potential legal hassles.

Rather than allowing someone to control me or force me to respond violently, I simply will move around the guy with hands stretched out, palms visible at the threshold distance, and walk away. If he goes for it, I already have him. And if he doesn't go for it, then it does not bother me in the least whatever he shouts out at me as I walk away down the street and continue with my life (such as, "You better keep moving, asshole " or "I'll pound your raggedy ass into the street, dickhead!").

My suggestion to you, dear reader, is to practice this "being alert, relaxed and letting it slide" approach as seriously and as often as you do the "come see the stars" technique. This gives you a choice and, with some experience and a rational mind, it's real easy to make the correct choice.

But first you have to provide yourself with options and, frankly, that is the real essence of self-defense training—providing yourself with some options. The correct option, when available, is to select the strategy of "offering no enemy," avoiding violence and its associated legal and medical problems. To do this, some people have to work on their fear of being seen as not being "real men" (that is, of not accepting the challenge of the woofer). In truth, this is nothing more than adolescent thinking and must be overcome. If you suffer from this affliction, first ask yourself this question: is it that you are afraid other people might think less of you for not fighting, or is it primarily that you are afraid that you will think less of yourself for not fighting? Either way, realize that the problem is that you are afraid. Overcoming our fear is job one in developing effective self-defense ability. Violence is almost always the product of fear. Don't allow yourself to be afraid and you can avoid a lot of unnecessary violence.

Drive-By Shooters

Currently, in Los Angeles and other mega-cities, it appears fashionable among some to drive their cars around carrying guns and to shoot people, apparently at random. Now, you might say, "How does all this philosophy apply to shit like that? Where's the interview there?"

Glad you asked.

First, consider why someone would do such a thing— drive by in a car at night to shoot and kill a stranger? Where's the payoff? What do they get out of it? The answer is, nothing.

Being desperate, feeling powerless and even voiceless in the environment they are born into, they perceive their own lives as essentially worthless. Now, feeling that their own lives are essentially worthless, how much more worthless is anybody else's? The answer is completely worthless. Thus, they don't hesitate to shoot anybody, and for no reason at all, as a means to express their personal desperation.

But, as their minds are warped, they have been defeated before they begin. Soon, they too will be the victims of this senseless cycle of slaughter. If you care to review the statistics for certain gangs in Los Angeles (for example), you will discover that the life expectancy of "shooters" is surprisingly brief. Tragically, though, before they stop some hot lead themselves, these gang bangers' promiscuous blasting away will claim the lives and spines of all too many innocent bystanders.

Do you see that the drive-by shooter displays the ultimate cowardice that is common to all bully types to some degree? In the drive-by shooter's case, his fear is so great that he fires a gun from inside a moving steel cage . . . from the darkness of a city night.

I don't have the hard data to back it up, but I imagine that even in a drive-by shooting the cretins pass by some people and, by some obtuse "logic" of the moment, pick out others as victims.

Now, let me add that while I was in L.A. teaching a class and talking with some cops, one of the officers told me about a suspect who was arrested when a drive-by shooting went down. In his confession he described how they spotted the potential victims walking on the sidewalk and then went around the block twice, scoping them out before they opened fire on their third pass. Now, why would they do this? Why did they have to go around the block three times to scope out the victims before they opened fire? It was not to identify the "proper" victims; this was a random shooting. Their going around the corner twice before actually doing the shooting was their form of the interview.

Even with the seemingly random violence of the drive-by shooter, awareness may still be your first and essential self-defense strategy. The aware person might notice the car, maybe even on the first pass. Then, instead of looking away (denying the threat), he might glance at the occupants. If he was really aware and had some luck, maybe he would perceive the gang bangers' intent or actually spot a weapon on that first pass. This would allow him to use the strategy of "offering no enemy" by simply not being on the street for pass number two. If he were a bit less alert, that first glance at the car might be just as the occupants began to stick their guns out the window to open fire. Still, even then, he would have a decent chance of avoiding being hit if he had mentally rehearsed this scenario in his mind before and determined how he might effect "target denial."

The whole idea is to be earlier and earlier on your perception of the potential threat and to have worked out beforehand how you will respond. This is not paranoia. Nor should this type of thinking disturb your enjoyment of a sunny day in the park. Think of it like looking both ways before you pull out in traffic or checking your rearview mirror before you pass somebody. Would you think of those actions as paranoia? No, they're only common-sense safe driving habits, and they occur almost at the preconscious level. You hardly even realize you are doing these things. Your basic self-defense strategies have to work the same way.

CHAPTER THREE

$60,000 to the Man Left Standing

Some of you good people (and, if you purchased this or my first book, then you are a good person) will recall that in my first book I talked about an imaginary contest where the winner would receive a significant amount of prize money in a *no-rules* hand-to-hand fight. This contest would be open to anyone, martial artists of any style, as well as street fighters and bouncers of "no style." The winner would be decided by who was left standing or by who surrendered.

I presented this imaginary contest to underscore some of the points I had raised in that book regarding martial art and martial arts technique in contrast with the realities of actual fighting and real-world violence.

Now, thanks in great part to Rorian Gracie and Mr. Art Davie (WOW Promotions), such a contest has come into existence. It is called the Ultimate Fighting Championship (UFC), and you can see it on Pay Per View or cable TV. Or you can buy videos of the previous battles. Alternatively, visit the next city it's held in and see it live.

The theme of this extraordinary contest, which pays the winner $60,000, is "Once Again, There Are No Rules." By the time you read this, the money might even be more than 60K. Hence, you gotta know some really tough guys show up for a payday like that. Yet, in truth, I don't think any of these fighters are there just for the money.

Also, by the time you read this, I think it's possible that the UFC will become a big enough money-making property that it might be sold and then called something else. In any case, let's hope it maintains its original raw beauty and does not degenerate into just another "tough-man" contest.

THE GRACIE BROTHERS

The UFC was organized by the Gracie brothers, a large family of legendary Brazilian jujutsu men. They call their system Gracie jujutsu and have always been willing to take on all comers. That means anyone—boxers, karate people, other jujutsu men, sumo wrestlers, kung fu and ninjutsu people, or aliens from outer space.

On occasion, people would show up at Rorian Gracie's dojo in Los Angeles to take up the challenge. These "fights" are videotaped, and Rorian (pronounced "Horian") once showed me some of these tapes. None of the challengers succeeded; none even came close as far as I could see.

The Gracies are grapplers. They close on their opponent, grapple with him, take him to the mat, and then it's "welcome to Gracie world." If you have no knowledge of their ground fighting, you are worse than helpless against a Gracie-trained fighter. They either will choke you to unconsciousness (if you don't tap out to surrender), or they will put you in a pain-compliance technique where you must "tap out" or you will pass out, unless your bones break first.

I know a very tough professional fighter, and to say that this guy is not the type to surrender is an understatement in the extreme. But I saw him surrender under a Gracie pain-compliance hold in the UFC.

The striking arts people—karate, kung fu, whatever—somehow convince themselves that they won't be taken to the ground. But every time they fight with the Gracie clan, they are taken to the ground and then it's all over.

In fact, from some of the Gracie challenge fights I saw on video (not the big-money UFC fights), it appeared clear to me that the Gracie fighter was toying with the challenger. I saw the Gracie man put one choke or joint technique after another on the challenger, only to release it and go to another hold without really applying the previous technique to its conclusion. In other words, he would put a choke on the guy that could end the fight right there, but then he would not choke him out. He would just flow into another fight-ending hold from which there was no possibility of escape. It was as if the Gracie man was saying, " . . . or I could knock him out like this . . . or like this . . . or maybe like this."

To let everyone know that his opponent was fighting as hard as he could, the Gracie fighter would often slap the challenger's face as he worked him over on the mat. As Rorian explained it to me, this was to demonstrate that the challenger, though fighting with all his heart and power, was completely helpless against the Gracie system, otherwise he would never tolerate such humiliation.

The Gracie strategy is based on the reality that very, very few fighters can drop a person with a single blow when that person is rushing in on them to achieve the grapple. Then, once the clinch occurs, the striking arts people have no leverage for a blow. Consequently, their hitting power is of no use to them. Rorian told me, "Hey, we don't claim to be punch-proof." I believe he meant that while it is possible that they could be knocked out while closing, this is an extremely unlikely outcome because it would require a one-punch KO on them.

The Gracies protect themselves very well on the way

in, and they don't telegraph much of anything. I'm still waiting to see that one-punch KO occur in one of these fights, but my honest feeling is that I'll have to wait a very long time. Though it is certainly possible that they could be knocked out just like Rorian said, the odds—and I think the skill and knowledge—are with the Gracies at this point.

In one sense, the Gracies' Ultimate Fighting contest exploits the naive training methods of other martial arts that, for the most part, pay very little attention to ground fighting. But, at least in the beginning of these contests, the Gracies also cleverly exploited the overconfidence that striking art people have in their techniques.

Is the Gracie System the Ultimate Self-Defense Art?

Almost needless to say, anyone with the guts and heart to step up to the Ultimate Fighting challenge has a good hold on proper combat attitude. But does this mean the Gracie system of jujutsu is the ultimate or most effective system of self-defense?

Well, as far as *ground fighting* is concerned, the Gracies' performance in these no-holds-barred contests provides us with good evidence that it is. In fact, now all the contestants have undertaken to learn some Brazilian jujutsu or other grappling art simply so they can have some chance to compete in the UFC. But consider this— there is more to a real fight than ground fighting or even technique itself, and no athletic contest can truly simulate a real fight as it occurs in the real world, *even in the absence of any rules.*

Now, why do I say this?

Because when two fighters step into the ring, they both know why they are there. They know they are there to fight, and each intends to win. This means they are perceptually ready for a fight, both in mind and body. On the other hand, in a real fight, *only* the assailant knows that he plans to attack, and he is not looking for a "fight" or any kind of contest. He is looking for an ambush . . . or even an execution.

RELYING ON THE PREDICTABLE RESPONSES OF THE ENEMY TO TRAP HIS DEFENSE

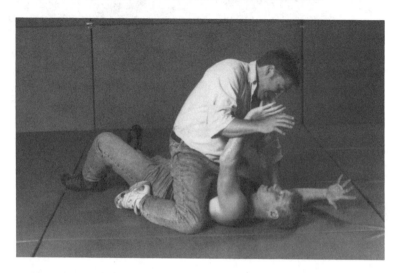

Having assumed the mounted position, I strike down at the enemy's head with my right hand while my left has pinned his right arm to the ground. He can only block my strike with his left hand now, and most people will do just that. At this point, my strike has been blocked.

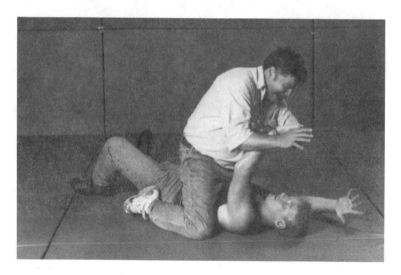

However, anticipating that he will block my strike in this manner, I am perceptually ready to catch his blocking arm immediately with my left hand.

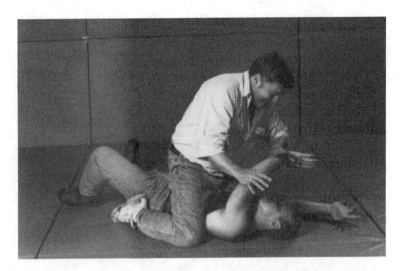

Note that an instant later my left hand has slid down toward his wrist while my right hand, palm down, controls his elbow. I am pushing down on his arm and drawing it across his body at the same time.

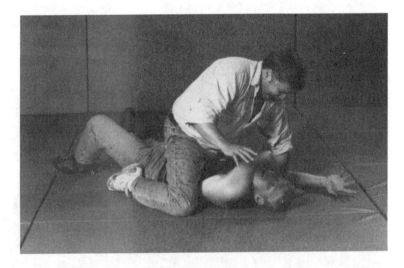

Even if the enemy was stronger, it would be very difficult for him to prevent my pushing his arm down and across his body in this manner. Not only do I have gravity on my side, but I am able to use both arms against his one. Once my hand touches the ground, it has "pinned" his left hand to the ground.

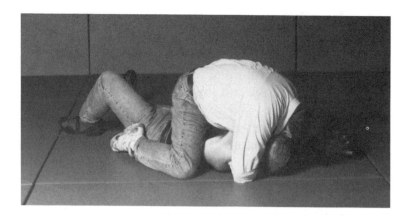

Now, to prevent the possibility of being thrown off myself, I lower my center of gravity as I pass his own left hand behind his neck and then capture it with my right hand.

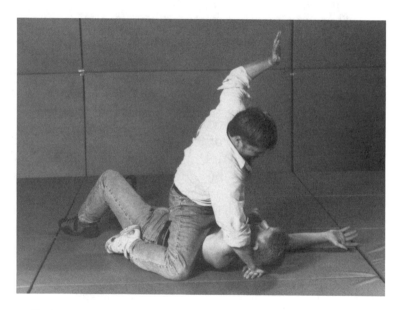

Having passed his left hand behind his neck and then captured it with my right hand, I have rendered the enemy all but helpless. Neither arm is available to him to check or block my strikes with my left hand. It would also be possible for me to draw a weapon at this point since he is immobilized and could not prevent same. During this entire sequence I would be vulnerable to attack by a second assailant.

Note that if I made my initial strike (fig. 4) with my left hand, I would end up with my trapping hand being my left and would thus be striking with my right hand in Figure 6.

If the assailant thought it would become a "contest" where he might get hurt or, in some cases, just suffer the indignity of losing, then most times he simply would not attack. As I explained in detail in the first book, the bully or aggressor is not looking for a fight; he's looking for a *victim*.

As for the intended victim (depending on his or her awareness and avoidance skills), most times he only realizes that he is in a fight after he takes that first sucker shot and sees that purple star pattern against the black background as his vision begins to clear. Many times, of course, that first sucker shot is followed immediately by another and another (continuous attack), and the victim never has a chance to defend himself at all, regardless of any martial training he might have.

Therefore, no athletic contest can simulate these very important and often decisive realities that exist in a real street fight.

Further, the Ultimate Fighting Championship is a one-on-one affair without the use of any weapons. A guy with a knife or a decent stick man would present a real problem for the Gracie one-on-one grappling fighting style—in the prize ring or in the street. But, then again, if the Gracie man had a stick or knife too, it could be a real horror show. Brutal as these Brazilians can sometimes be in the prize ring, my impression is that if they had to fight for real it would make their prize ring work look like a body massage in a fancy health club. Further, if attacked with a knife I definitely don't think they would grapple. Rather, they would deal with it altogether differently, and most likely their assailant would get the point. Still, I have to say that the Gracie system, strong as it is, is not applicable to fighting someone with a knife or for fighting more than one person at a time.

Rorian Gracie acknowledged this, but quite reasonably asked my companion (a strong fighter), "Do you think you could defeat two assailants that had your skill and experience in any case?" Now, I feel I must expand on Rorian's thought and point out that in a real fight the

WEAPONS HAVE ALWAYS BEEN THE FIRST CHOICE FOR COMBAT, SO BE ALERT FOR THEM!

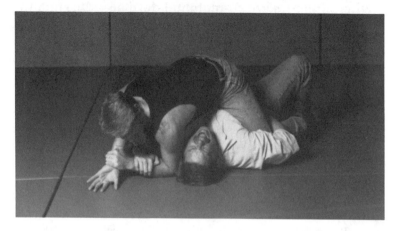

Here I am being held down in a figure 4 lock. As my enemy raises my elbow off the ground, it places painful pressure on my elbow joint and can dislocate my arm from its socket if done powerfully and violently by a strong enough adversary. Although my right hand is still free, I cannot get leverage to land a blow with any real power, nor can I reach any sensitive targets. The assailant has a good chance to control me through pain compliance by increasing the pressure on my arm.

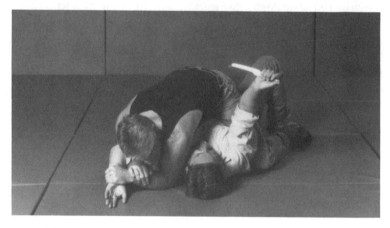

YIKES! I have a solution to this dilemma. The knife changes everything. While I can't strike a powerful enough blow to be damaging with my bare hands, the knife will be deadly at once. The assailant has failed to protect himself from the appearance of the weapon with this technique. Here I have a large blade, but any knife, no matter how small, will do the trick in this situation. A small pocket pistol could be used here as well.

combatants are almost never equal in skill and experience. Indeed, this only happens in an athletic contest, where fighters are so-matched deliberately, such that there can be an interesting contest. Certainly I agree with Rorian that it is very difficult to fight more than one person, but I also feel it might be much harder to do in an athletic contest (prize fight) than in an actual battle.

Again, this is because of the differences between a real fight and any fighting contest. The assailants who attack for real are not prepared for you to take the fight to them; they are not prepared to get hurt and keep fighting. On top of this, real fights do not occur in a prize ring, and weapon potential is always at hand outside that sterile environment (unfortunately, your assailants can be armed as well).

To underscore this idea briefly, I shall convey the following tale. Three people once attacked me by ambush after they had fractured the skull of my pal with a stick when we walked outside a door into the parking lot. Fortunately, they used no knives. Why did they not draw knives? Again, because they thought it would all go their way. They never imagined anything else would happen but that they would take us by surprise and beat us to death or at least break a lot of our bones using the stick and their boots.

As it happened, all three of them ended up in the hospital that night, and it was they who had multiple fractures and lacerations that had to be sewed up. Not to digress too far with this tale, I'll simply say that though they hit me more times than I connected with them, my blows were always more damaging. Also, I used a parked car as an environmental weapon when I beat their heads against the sharp edge of the rain gutter of the car's roof.

Now, suppose it were a prize ring and these same three guys were given six weeks or so to train for the fight. Would I do as well? The correct answer is, probably not. Because if they showed up they would more likely be psychologically prepared for a fight, not just ready to ambush us like they tried that night.

But again, even though there were three of them, and even if they had not already had the experience of the parking lot fight, do you think they would have been willing to step up to such a prize fight against both me and my pal? Again, the correct answer is, no, not likely. Experiment with this idea—it's a significant one about the nature and mind of these people.

It's said that a picture is worth a thousand words. Well, there are 30 pictures per second in a video image, so watch a video of the UFC. It says a lot about the limitations of martial arts and their techniques in a contest that, thus far, best simulates some important *physical* aspects of a real fight.

After you see one of these Ultimate Fighting contests, you may wonder how anyone could really think, "Yeah, but a good TKD man (or kung fu man, ninjutsu man, boxer, etc.) could beat them." The fact is that people primarily believe what they wish to believe, which is simply what they feel they need to believe, even when the truth of the matter is stuck right in front of their faces.

THE IMPORTANCE OF THE TRAINING METHOD

In Gracie jujutsu, one learns the holds, takedowns, and so on by doing them with an opponent who fully resists and has a knowledge of the same system. This is one of the real strengths of the Gracie system: the *training method itself.*

People are brought along step by step in the Gracie system, just like in most any other martial art. But the important difference here is, the Gracie system teaches you to grapple by allowing you to grapple. In a striking art, you really can't train like that. You can't learn to break someone's clavicle by actually breaking someone's clavicle in the dojo.

The big problem with the classic karate or TKD approach in teaching striking technique is simply that one cannot strike dynamically and with full power on the unprotected opponent. Hence, because of the training method, karate people may fail to learn how to strike with full power, and they may never know it until their first real fight.

Any system that can use a training method that is almost the same as the actual employment of the techniques in a true combat situation has an overpowering advantage over one that cannot.

In his *Tao of Jeet Kune Do*, Bruce Lee put it this way: "The best preparation for an event is the event itself."

Why Does the Karate Fighter So Often Fear the Boxer?

I don't want to waste too much ink on this; hence, I offer it as a discoverable fact that many karate people have a fear that the guy they may have to fight for real may train as a boxer. This is because the karate person fears that he would most likely be beaten by a boxer.

Of course, there are also plenty of karate-trained people who don't have enough sense to fear the boxer. This is not really a problem with their intelligence, it is simply a lack of information and experience that leads a karate black belt to imagine a boxer would be no problem for him. "Why, shucks," he reasons, "I'd just side-step that boxer's punch and take out a knee."

Still, many karate guys often secretly fear that "head hunter" boxer with a pair of fast hands . . . and rightfully so. But why? After all, every technique in the boxing art is also present in a complete karate curriculum. Even Chuck Norris will throw a left jab and a cleaner version of the old "John Wayne" hook that we all know and love so well. All the hand techniques in boxing exist in karate, though they may be greatly deemphasized because of karate's sport nature.

So if it is not the *techniques* of boxing that the karate man worries about, what is it? The answer is all but self-evident: at the root of what the karate man fears is the boxing *training method*. The boxer is used to hitting people in the head full force and taking a few head shots himself, but the karate stylist most often has had no such training experience.

You learn to box by boxing. From the first day in boxing, you put on gloves and headgear and actually box. It's contact training; you take shots that rattle your brain, and you dish out the same as best you are able. On the other hand, you can study karate for years and never hit anybody or really get hit yourself.

As you might expect, the boxing training method weeds out the dilettantes quickly, since these types give up boxing after the first day or so . . . if they ever show up in the gym in the first place.

An Effective Training Method Must Allow the Student to Discover and Exercise His Warrior Spirit

It would be easy to say that the people who quit boxing training early just don't "have the heart" for a real scrap. But I don't think it's necessarily that simple.

The problem for some is that the boxing training method fails to provide them with the experience of a situation and environment that would allow them to discover their true survival spirit—that is, what they have deep inside and have not, as yet, truly experienced.

I submit that everyone has the survival imperative inside them. It exists on the "frog" brain level and not in the superconscious mind. (Something that exists in our superconscious mind occupies our immediate thoughts at a particular moment; it is the focus of our attention.) This is why tai chi people will talk directly about engaging the "reptilian brain" for combat. Therefore, since everyone does have at least latent warrior spirit, one of the first objectives of an effective self-defense training program must be to actualize that warrior spirit in the student by allowing him to execute techniques with full power on a live, moving assailant under adrenal stress, just as those techniques would be used in actual combat. This means allowing students to *experience* their warrior spirit and thus recognize their power.

For some, boxing serves well in this capacity, but many others quit very early in the boxing program and many more never get up the nerve to start. Consequently, while I rate the boxing training method as one of the best, I must also recognize that it's not suitable for everyone. This is primarily because boxing assumes a certain level of "heart" and "warrior spirit" from day one. Unfortunately, our mainstream society works hard at socializing people to deny or ignore their warrior spirit. Therefore, boxing can be just too much too fast for a lot of people. But again, this does not mean that these people have no warrior spirit, or, as it is sometimes miscalled, "killer instinct."

Secondarily, and on the technical side, there is also the problem in boxing of striking with the closed fist to the head, which, for most people, will mean broken bones in the hand in a real fight. Boxers wear gloves and tape their hands carefully to prevent this and, even so, occasionally even professional boxers still break bones in their hands. But this is a minor technical issue compared to the previously addressed concern.

Proper combat attitude requires that one be in touch with his warrior spirit. Therefore, since proper combat attitude is more important than polished technique, it follows that, in a given training method, *if* we were forced to choose between better actualizing the warrior spirit or better imparting skill in physical technique, we would have to choose the former. Of course, this assumes we are training our students to survive a street attack rather than win a martial arts tournament (regardless of the tournament's rules, lack of same, or contact level).

On the Path to Developing a More Effective Self-Defense Training Method

Obviously, if the student is to strike with full power to the most vulnerable targets on the human body, and since his "target" must be a living, moving "assailant," we are going to need some type of padding or protection, at least for the assailant in our training program. Yet when we look at the existing model of boxing, which uses padded hands (boxing gloves) and protective headgear to allow full-contact fighting, we can see that this method apparently begins on too accelerated a track for many people. Further, recognizing how real-world attacks develop, and having observed the modus operandi of real-world assailants (as detailed in my video *Self-Defense against the Sucker Puncher)*, we must teach a lot more than technique. An effective self-defense program must condition the student to control and channel fear and to control the disabling effects of adrenal stress.

In short, the training method must condition the student to recognize the cues that precede the potential attack (the interview stages) and, rather than deny or ignore these cues, employ them collectively as the stimulus that switches their consciousness from the denial mode of normal, civilized behavior to a full but reasonably relaxed focus on the threat. This facilitates the transition to frog brain work should it come to actual combat. However, since this involves awareness, it also makes possible the *avoidance* of most battles in the first place. Remember, avoidance of the conflict is always everyone's best survival strategy (and I mean *every time*, people). Avoidance is the very essence of real-world self-defense.

Finally, if the attack is already in progress, or if the avoidance strategy is failing, the student must recognize this and be able to enter and strike down his enemy without hesitation and without restraint. This reality must include preemptive striking when it is clear that the actual physical attack is imminent.

Over the last five years since I wrote *Bouncer's Guide to Barroom Brawling,* I have been working on a program that addresses these very issues. Since that time we have put more than a few hundred people through the course.

Admittedly, should the meek inherit the earth, yours truly may come up pitifully short on real estate holdings, but I will tell you frankly that this training method works far better than I ever imagined was possible.

Further, I will go so far as to say that this method has never failed to increase a person's self-defense potential quite significantly, regardless of whether he or she has had any previous self-defense training or none at all. I do not pretend to have invented this method; frankly, I don't think anyone can reasonably make any such claim. The method is an evolution and synthesis of many individuals' talents, experience, and vision.

However, I am arrogant enough to believe that I have made a significant contribution to the evolution of this training method, as have others (not least of all being Mike Haynack; Mark Morris; "the Professor," Mike Belzer; Bill Kipp; Tom Rodriguez; Ronsky; Jeff Chean; Melissa Soalt; Randy Miamarro; and others that I have had the privilege to work with in this effort).

In the following chapters I will present the methodology of this training program, the logic upon which it is predicated, and how it addresses the core problems in preparing someone to deal with the real-world problems of an actual self-defense encounter (such as I identified and pontificated on for 269 pages in my first book).

CHAPTER FOUR

Scenario-Based Training

The essence of the applied self-defense training technology that we employ (and at this point I think it is reasonable to call it a technology) is the adrenal stress of the fight scenario. (Once again, I remind you that I make no claim to having originated this method, nor do I think anyone reasonably can, but most likely you have little interest in how it started anyway, so I will not try your patience with all that now.)

In a fight scenario, the fighter (in some programs called the "student") is given instructions such as, "Your objective is to walk to the far side of the mat and then pass through the two air shields you see over there. The air shields represent a doorway. You may encounter problems; deal with them appropriately." We call this the "portal of safety" scenario.

As the fighter begins his walk, the "Bulletman"

(armored assailant) appears, and his behavior will be unpredictable. The Bulletman may act friendly, or he make act mentally deranged. He might be verbally threatening, or he may just attack immediately without any warning or woof at all.

The point is that the fighter has no advanced knowledge of what will happen in the scenario. He or she must adapt and deal with whatever goes down during that scenario.

THE CRITICAL ROLE OF THE BULLETMAN

The man who gets into the armor and plays the part of the assailant, the Bulletman, is the key instructor in the course. He is not just a moving heavy bag that the fighter pounds on.

A good Bulletman is truly a master instructor, and there are very few martial artists, or anyone else, who can rise to the challenge of getting into that armor and doing the job well.

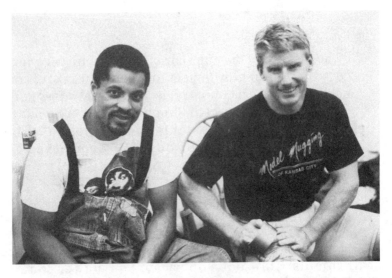

Master Bulletmen Mr. Thomas Rodriguez on the left and Mr. Bill Kipp on the right. It takes a lot of stamina and skill to get into the padded armor and do the job right. The Bulletman is the heart of the adrenal stress scenario-based training method.

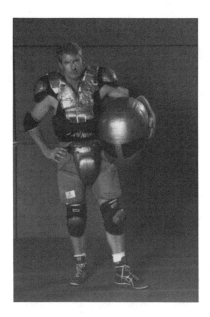

Bill Kipp displays the basic armor of the Bulletman. Each suit is custom-fitted to the individual and costs about $1,200 to fabricate. The head gear contains a professional football helmet inside. The groin protector is made partly of semirigid plastics and foam. Mr. Mark Morris is the premier designer of this equipment. The armor, tough as it is, cannot do the job alone. The man inside must know how to take the shots without being injured. He does this by "rolling with the shots" and by perceiving the blow. The more skillful the fighters become—and this happens pretty quickly in this training method—the more difficult the Bulletman's job becomes and the more hard shots he absorbs.

The Bulletman must have a sense of what ability level the fighter is at, and then he must attack in a manner that continues to challenge that fighter's ability. Sometimes this means offering the perfect opportunity for the fighter to make the perfect strike, and sometimes it means tackling the fighter from behind while he is standing in line.

The armor does not protect the Bulletman completely; he must have the athletic and martial skill to protect himself by reading body cues and "rolling with the punches," so to speak. He must also rely on the instructors with the whistles to stop the scenario when he is "knocked out." Without good Bulletmen, there is no scenario training program; therefore, it's essential that they not be disabled in the fight scenarios.

Moreover, the quality of the scenario-based instruction itself depends chiefly on the quality of the Bulletmen in the suits. Since the armor cannot protect the Bulletman against some types of attack techniques, even though these attacks might be real useful in an actual fight, they are too dangerous and therefore are not used in the fight scenario simulations. But, while the armor has some limitations, the primary limitation to this training method is the scarcity of people with the skill, spirit, and character that are demanded to put on that armor and then use it effectively as an instructor. This limitation to the scenario-based training method overshadows any other by far.

Physical Limitations of the Armor

The types of techniques that cannot be used in the fight scenarios because the armor cannot adequately protect the Bulletman against them include kicks to the knees, joint locks, and joint lock throws, such as are found in the aikido, akijutsu, or jujutsu. In addition, most "use of the environment" techniques, such as breaking the opponent's balance and then actually running him into a solid object such as a wall or post, cannot be executed against the Bulletman in the fight scenarios.

Finally, there are some martial arts people who, after they have done two or three of the fight scenarios, become capable of landing shots that basically just get through the armor because of their raw power, proper focus, and correct chamber of depth. Most often these people weigh close to 200 pounds (though some are much smaller), and many times they are black belts in a striking art like karate or TKD.

When a shot gets through the armor like this, it takes a lot out of the Bulletman. Without the armor, he might have been killed, but even with it he sustains an unacceptable level of trauma or an actual concussion.

As a side note, observing large black belts develop this hitting capacity in the fight scenarios shows me that, while unlikely, the old karate theme (particularly in reference to the Okinawan karate) i.e., "one strike, one kill," is at least a true possibility.

Commonly Asked Questions
about the Bulletman's Role

First let me say that two fundamental questions I list here are asked exclusively by people who have not taken the course. I cannot recall anyone who has observed (or even studied a video of) this training method asking these questions, and no one has ever phrased them quite as rudely as I do here, but I wish to be frank for clarity.

Question # 1: "Come on, the guy comes out in that Pillsbury-Dough-Boy suit, barks out some shit, and then stands there while the student pounds on him. He doesn't really fight back, and besides, the student always knows he's going to 'win.' How can that develop anything but a dangerous sense of false confidence in the student?"

Even if the assumptions in this question were all true (which they are not), ask yourself, might this scenario method still be an improvement on, or a very worthwhile addition to, the traditional Asian method of training, where the student never gets woofed on and never hits anybody either?

Further, as far as instilling a dangerous sense of false confidence in the student, the traditional Asian method can scarcely be beat on that score. Many black belts assume without question that they know how to fight, when, in fact, they don't even really know what a fight is (maybe they haven't even ever *seen* one).

On balance, though, it's apparent to me that the Asian methods and techniques have value and so does the scenario training method. When both are used together, students are provided with a much more effective self-defense program, and their chances of survival are increased markedly.

In response to the idea that "the Bulletman doesn't really fight back; he just stands there while the student pounds on him," this is simply not true. That is not how we do it.

The Bulletman responds according to the individual fighter's skill level. Some people are "paralyzed" with fear in the scenarios, just as they would be in the street. These people need a successful experience before they can break out of this paralysis. In this case, the Bulletman will offer the easy targets and may over-respond to the actual power of a strike. This is sometimes a necessary step in getting the student to start thinking like and thus moving like a fighter. With each new scenario, the fighter faces a Bulletman who is more evasive in his movements and faster in his own attacks—in short, who challenges the student based on what level the student is at.

As far as the idea that the Bulletman does not actually strike the student/fighter, in my program the Bulletman often will. In a few rare cases I have even told the Bulletman to give the student a tasty head shot right off the bat (as in, "snap his head back a bit") because the student needed this to achieve the necessary adrenalization effect or to get past a denial response. On the other hand, for the confident, experienced, and trained fighter, we pull out all kinds of slimy tricks because it is necessary to instill some fear in this class of fighter. The course cannot achieve its full objective if the fighter does not experience some level of fear and confusion.

This is why we will sometimes have a second Bulletman attack the fighter from behind while the student is being woofed on by the first Bulletman. Another personal favorite is having the Bulletman tackle the fighter from behind while he is totally absorbed in watching someone else's fight scenario. Other "surprise treats" include the Bulletman's concealing a towel behind his back and then throwing it in the fighter's face. This confuses the fighter and obscures his vision just as the Bulletman attacks with the blade.

Surprise weapons such as the knife, stick, or even a pistol will come up in a basics class (which otherwise is not a weapons class) in order to adrenalize the experienced fighters faster and to force them to adapt, move, and deal with it.

If the fighter begins to enter into flailing behavior or otherwise gets into a position where the Bulletman's attack is prevailing, then the scenario is stopped and the fighter is given another scenario to correct his mistake. This is important because the adrenal conditioning is strong, and we must avoid conditioning mistakes into fighters. We are not training them to lose; we are training them to win.

However, we need to be objective if we are to improve on any program. At present we are working on a lighter limited armor for the fighter so that, in more advanced classes, the Bulletman can strike surprise shots on the fighter with more juice. This will help the fighter learn to take a stiff shot and still keep fighting and still protect himself.

Boxing accomplishes this. But it would be a real mistake to pad up the fighter so that the scenarios became like two boxers sparing with head gear and gloves in an athletic match. We are not training people to spar. We are training people to enter and strike down the enemy. We are training people to win a street fight, not an athletic contest.

This is not to detract from the boxing training method, because it is a pretty good one. Boxing does involve hard contact on a moving aggressor. But the scenario training is more effective and more accessible to most people from a strict applied-self-defense point of view.

Our scenario-based training method is sometimes referred to as "asymmetric" training. Consider what this concept means.

In symmetric training methods such as boxing, both combatants are trying to win; that is, beat the other. In contrast, in asymmetric training methods, one combatant, the instructor in the armored suit, is not trying to "defeat" the student fighter; he is training him or her to hit hard and effectively.

In the symmetric training scenario, the boxers do not have to make any decisions on when it is appropriate (legally, tactically, etc.) to attack—the fight is on the minute they step into the ring.

But making such decisions under the stress of the woof and interview—that is, knowing when violence is necessary or, more simply put, knowing when it's time to "go off" and then just stepping up and doing it—is a very important (often decisive) aspect of a real self-defense situation. It is where most people have their greatest problem. Asymmetric scenario-based training forces the fighter to experience and overcome this fundamental problem.

Question #2: "When I see video of the fight scenarios, like in your light-force knockout video, *Blitzkrieg*, it seems I see only three or four techniques ever being used, and the fights seem all 'one way' once the Bulletman takes the first hard shot. How come?"

Because that's the way real fights go. Once the Bulletman takes a solid shot that he judges would knock him out or stun him into semiconsciousness for a moment, he responds in a realistic fashion. You may have observed in the videos that some of the hand or elbow strikes to the Bulletman's head actually knock his feet off the ground. Think what effect such a strike would have on an unprotected assailant.

After such a blow, consider what the knee-to-the-head strike would do to an unarmored person actually raising himself up off the pavement. It would certainly end the fight and, in some cases, it would kill or permanently injure the person. In fact, Bulletmen have been knocked out through the armor by the knee strike, and in one case a Bulletman's jaw was broken. By the way, the Bulletman's helmet includes at its core a professional football player's helmet. Yet these helmets have actually been damaged in fight scenarios. The Bulletman whose jaw was broken was struck by a knee to the head by a woman weighing less than 145 pounds with no previous training. Actually, the Bulletman often takes what would be two or three shots that would knock out an unprotected human being before he goes down.

I must point out that the most often heard report from both male and female students who were later attacked for real in the street is, "It was a lot easier than the Bulletman; the guy just lay there after the first shot."

Real fights are most often one-way affairs once a good, stunning blow is landed and then followed up on immediately (continuous attack). After all, this is the sucker puncher's whole game—make that first shot good and then keep blasting so the victim has no chance to recover. On the unaware victim, this sucker puncher strategy generally works pretty well, too.

As far as only a limited number of techniques being used in the fights, this too is by design. You simply don't need a whole repertoire of martial arts techniques for a real street fight. What you need are maybe two or three shots that you can deliver with disabling force and the mind-set to continue the attack until the enemy is incapable of coming back or posing any threat to you at all.

I reiterate—any knowledge or skill in physical technique is irrelevant in a real fight if it is not accompanied by proper combat attitude and mind-set. The adrenal stress conditioning of the fight scenarios is not only a very powerful tool in showing people this reality, it is also a very powerful tool in developing proper combat attitude itself.

THE ROLE OF THE FIGHTER

Avoidance

In response to the Bulletman's actions, the fighters' first self-defense strategy is always avoidance. They may elect to do this nonverbally through their body posture, movement, gaze, etc. Alternatively, they may talk to the Bulletman, either to set a "boundary," or to gather further insight into the Bulletman's true intentions as they demonstrate that they are not intimidated or frozen with fear.

The fighters know they must always keep track of the Bulletman's hands, because the Bulletman might draw a weapon at anytime. At the same time, the fighters must not allow their vision to "tunnel in" on the Bulletman, because this would make them vulnerable, particularly to the surprise attack by a possible second Bulletman assailant.

Neither can the fighters go off prematurely, that is, attack preemptively without justifiable and reasonable cause. The opening of the scenario, the interview phase by the Bulletman, conditions the fighters to control themselves under stress. They learn to relax their minds and control their breathing under the adrenal stress of the interview scenario.

As I said earlier, many potential assailants will give up their idea of attacking if confronted with a person who, subjected to their woof, still remains focused and relaxed. The reason relaxed behavior on the part of the intended victim during the woofing worries the aggressor is that he is now dealing with the unknown and the unfamiliar. In short, the woofer fears that he may become the victim if he picks on a dog that bites. The whole point of the interview is to first discover whether the potential victim may be too dangerous to attack and then to instill fear in the potential victim to impair his ability to defend himself.

Indeed, if the fighter in the training scenario handles his deescalation or avoidance skills particularly well, then the Bulletman may not attack at all. In such a case,

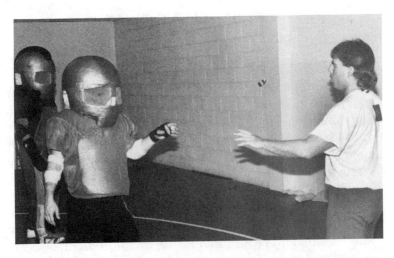

Here a fight scenario begins with the woof. The fighter attempts to deescalate and avoid a fight by derailing the interview. Facing two potential assailants can be very unnerving. The scenario gives the fighter a chance to practice "showing no fear" and shutting down the interview. Sometimes the Bulletmen will attack, but if the fighter's projection and spirit seem strong enough to the Bulletman, they may choose to let him pass without a fight. The fighter never knows what's going to happen, just like real life.

the fighter later gets a scenario where avoidance is not possible and there is a fight.

Some Lessons from My Bouncer Days

When I first started working as a bouncer (an economic necessity at that time), I'd been in a few street fights and had studied various martial arts to reasonably advanced levels for more than 15 years. At age 26 I was in good physical condition and likely had a bit of the "young buck" syndrome.

However, I believe that I was nearly always reasonable and polite to people, at least at their woof stage. But due to the times, the culture of the Wild West, and that uranium "boom town" mentality, there were fights most every night I worked as a bouncer. Fights were the norm.

Since I covered most of these barroom war stories in *A Bouncer's Guide to Barroom Brawling,* I don't want to digress too much from the immediate point by rehashing those. Suffice it to say that after three or four real fist fights, which included some pool cue- and bottles-and-boots-type battles, my chief impression was that the fights all seemed pretty uncontrolled, sloppy, and vicious. Although I was an experienced martial artist, rarely did I employ any but the most basic (if any) martial arts techniques. Things just happened too fast.

One evening after the place closed for the night, I can remember sitting at the bar with a drink in my left hand and my swollen right hand in a pitcher of ice water. I clearly remember asking myself whether I could or should continue with this work or just quit. Why I didn't quit then is not easy to explain, and some might argue was not a rational decision. But I stayed for a while and, remarkably even to me, I actually got somewhat used to people woofing on me real heavy, actually trying to set me up for some sort of ambush, or just going for that old reliable sucker punch. Dealing with that level of stuff became almost a reflex with me, like when a bartender wipes up a spill with the towel he perpetually keeps in his hand and never even looks down at the bar to do it.

(Okay, a bit of an exaggeration, but you get the idea.) Most of this level of aggressive stuff I learned to "short-circuit" so it never really went to a fight because the guy never attacked me.

That these guys would often back down was surprising to me at first, though I quickly came to rely on strategies for dealing with physically aggressive and threatening people in a way that avoided a physical battle. These strategies were based on my observations of the many woofers and sucker-punchers I had seen and an analysis of their modus operandi. After a while I realized that the woof was really the beginning of the fight and the easiest way to "win" was to derail the interview process.

Even back then it flashed through my mind that just about anybody could handle most of these tough guys (and without a fight most times) if they just had the right attitude and didn't allow themselves to get scared and rattled.

Basically (though not universally), these would-be assailants were dealing with some emotional pain or emotional disability that was at the true source of their aggressive behavior. Despite their physical appearance or aggressive verbal abuse and threats, in an important sense they were vulnerable to every bully's special kind of fear. It was true that these guys would not hesitate to sucker-punch or blindside someone or to woof him into a display of paralyzing fear before blasting him with the sucker shot. But most often they would back down when they thought they might have to deal with a person who they saw wasn't rattled and suspected might be ready for a fight.

Now here is the mental leap I want you to make. When it did come to a physical fight, I was still fighting that same kind of person. Very few fights ended with the assailant(s) unconscious on the floor or with injuries such that they could not continue to fight. Many times they stopped all aggressive activity after they took a few good shots or were thrown. This is because after that there was *nothing in it for them anymore*. Think about what this says about the woof being the start of the fight and why it is so important to one's self-defense ability to recognize and deal with the woof properly.

More and more in my bar work I began to experiment with ways to be earlier and earlier in my perception of the preparations a person might be making for an attack. Those attack preparations might be directed toward me, but most times they were directed toward someone else. Spotting them early saved me from having to fight a lot of guys. In some instances one could say that it was the *thought* of the preparation to attack that I first perceived.

Now, I'm not talking kung fu flute music and candles-burning-in-the-temple stuff here. I am saying that an intention in the mind is very often betrayed in the face and body. The game of poker is principally about reading the cards another person holds by the expressions on his face and other body cues. The saying "he had a poker face" means that a person has consciously concealed his thoughts or intentions, preventing them from being displayed on his face. Hell, consider the whole profession of acting—is it not often about communicating emotion, thought, and intentions without any spoken word or dialogue but only through facial expression, body carriage, and so on?

Deconditioning the Denial Response

There is a natural tendency in some good people to turn away from or deny a perceived evil intention on the part of another. This must be overcome, and it can be using scenario-based training. You cannot ignore your enemies, as this will encourage them to attack.

Being aware of the nature and objective of the woof and the nature of the woofer not only made fights more avoidable for me but gave me an edge on the assailant if he did attack. This is because I had denied him his opportunity to execute his regular modus operandi (a surprise attack). If he then attacked anyway, he did so with a more divided (less confident) mind.

Equally important, a potential assailant was much

more likely to betray or telegraph his attack with me standing right there waiting for it and *him knowing this*. Picture this in your mind. (I will stoop to using a Wild West paradigm, the Hollywood gunfighter scene.) Consider the scene where the bad guy woofs on the stranger by challenging, threatening, or insulting him in some way. After the obligatory period where the good guy may attempt to avoid violence, the good guy turns and faces the bad-guy gunfighter with a relaxed and confident expression on his face and says something like, "It's your play now, pilgrim."

The bad guy is either then shown wetting his lips in fear before he attempts to draw and is then killed, or he backs off, sometimes with a trailing woof as he leaves. Though mostly a romantic fantasy, I think this scene has some significant truths in it as well. Like a legend, the cliché often develops around some kernel of repeatedly observed truth.

You are cautioned, however—note that I am using words like "almost every time," or "generally," and so on. Yes, dear reader, there are bad guys out there who, when they wet their lips, do so in an anticipation of the joy and rush of the kill. They may draw their iron and blast a hole through you before you even clear leather. But happily, these types are few compared to the legions of woofers who will do all manner of injury to you, *but only if you let them*. Also, the really "hot guns" (truly dangerous psychos) often make themselves conspicuous by foreshadowing their special qualities if you are aware and attuned to same. Such discrimination is all but impossible if your mind is preoccupied by fear (adrenal effects).

Further, and I will not try to tell you otherwise, things like the size, height, weight, and the musculature of your potential assailant are always significant. Bigger guys generally do hit harder and are sometimes a lot harder to hurt even if you do land your best shot. But while size and weight are important, I would say that, in my observation, it is the psychological aspects of the fight (which begin with the earliest perception of the interview) that are often more decisive than size and weight, or, I might add, technical fighting skill, in determining the outcome of a real fight. In this ratio I include the many fights that never actually came to physical blows but certainly would have if the fighter had not handled the psychology of the interview effectively.

Striking Preemptively

Some scenarios may demand a preemptive strike from the fighter.

A preemptive strike is an attack (i.e., the striking of a blow) at a point in the interview process where the fighter has established in his or her own mind that an attack is either in progress or imminent This may occur while the Bulletman is still in the woofing stage of the interview.

To quote the "Little Dragon" (Bruce Lee) from *The Tao*

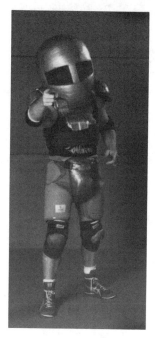

of Jeet Kune Do once again, "The best time to attack is on the enemy's preparation to attack."

This is certainly true; the trick is to recognize when the enemy is preparing to attack. Scenario training facilitates this by conditioning the fighter to recognize a woof for what it is (a probe by the aggressor to see if it's safe to attack) and to understand the steps in the progression of the interview.

Attacking with Full-Contact Striking

When the Bulletman attacks, the fight is on, and the student goes immediately to fighting at 100-percent plus intensity, striking the Bulletman with full power to the head, groin, neck, midsection, and so on. These fights will sometimes go to the

Helmet on but without his clothing concealing his basic armor, the Bulletman points and begins a woof on the camera.

The armor allows one to execute many techniques full-force on a moving, living "assailant." There is just no substitute for this in learning how to execute a technique well in a combat fashion. No holding back makes it easier and faster to learn how to do it and develops the all-essential confidence in fighters that allows them to just "step up and do it" when the situation demands it. Here we see a preemptive strike. The Bulletman has woofed and has stepped toward me reaching for a grab with his right hand.

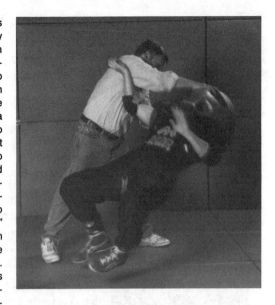

My left hand brushes the grabbing hand to the side as I step past the assailant immediately and blast him with the "alien from hell" technique. Note that his face is looking at the ceiling and the impact has knocked him off his feet. There are several sweet variations on this particular beauty. The "alien from hell" version is best applied on an enemy about your own height or shorter.

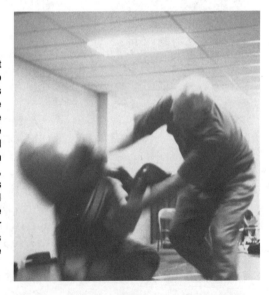

Battling "Joe," at age 72, is still taking no shit off anyone. This is a nice preemptive strike with the iron palm to the face. It knocks the Bulletman down and Joe is sticking with him for the finish-off. Mike, the Amazing Eagle, refs in the background and won't blow the whistle until Joe delivers two or three more solid shots on the Bulletman before his enemy can recover.

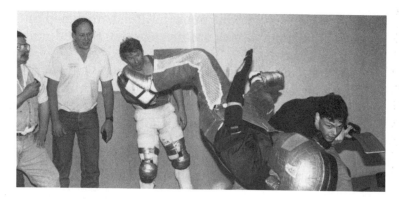

Notice the meat cleaver in the Bulletman's right hand. He never gets a chance to use it because the fighter has remained calm under the woof and avoids the adrenal effect of "tunnel vision." Hence he perceives the first motion the Bulletman makes to reach for something behind his back and enters on the enemy—in this case with a real tear-jerker of a technique, a "sumio tosh"-type throw.

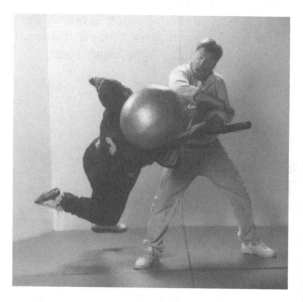

Here the Bulletman attacks with an overhead strike with a stick. However, he never gets the shot off because the instant he raises the weapon to chamber the strike, I enter on him and catch his weapon arm with my left and twist it down to my own center as I deliver the forearm strike to the head. The shot has very good power because the enemy's head is being drawn into the blow. Note the "torque" or twist in the Bulletman's body. The blow has knocked him off his feet such that for an instant he is "weightless"; the dominant force becomes the rotation that has been applied to his weapon arm. The forearm strike is a real sweetie. It is more powerful than a hand strike but must be executed very close to the assailant. The forearms can take a lot of impact without damage, but the hand is much more vulnerable to being busted on a person's hard skull. It doesn't always work this sweet in real life, but if you're shameless enough and take enough photos, you can get one like this too.

ground. The fighter continues the attack unabated until either the whistle blows or it is clear that the Bulletman is unconscious.

At that point the fighter makes a brief pat-down of the Bulletman for any weapons or secures for himself any weapon the Bulletman may have deployed during the fight, while continually glancing about for other potential assailants.

The fight is over when the fighter does these things and then escapes from the mat after the whistle has blown.

THE FIGHT SCENARIOS ENGAGE
INVOLUNTARY BIOCHEMICAL RESPONSES

Some people reading this book might think, "Shit, some guy in that Pillsbury-Dough-Boy suit barking at me from inside that huge helmet isn't going to bother me at all." Indeed, some people might even think that it would be "fun" to "beat up" on that guy in the rubber suit.

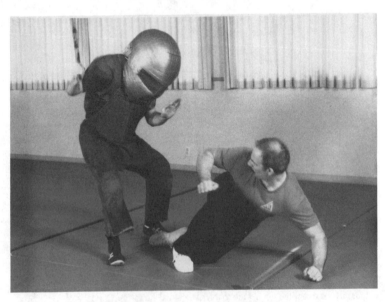

Here Dr. Al Tino gets the surprise rushing attack with the stick. He only has time to drop off the attack line as his left foot checks the assailant's foot, thus tripping him.

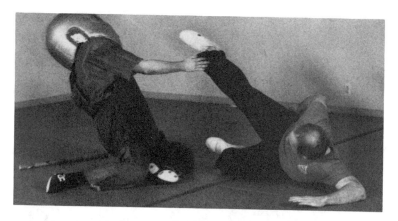

In this next photo, the Bulletman has been tripped, and as he tries to jump back up to continue the attack, the Doc gives him the old side kick to the face. Here we see the Bulletman's head snap back from the blow. Doc Al will continue to attack the Bulletman and recover the stick for himself.

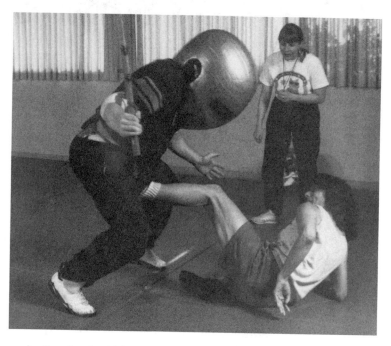

Another charging stick attack. This woman goes to the ground to avoid being hit and forces the Bulletman to come down to get her. But, it's the old thrust kick to the yarbles on a closing assailant. The blow will knock back the Bulletman's pelvis such that he falls straight down face-first. The fighter will continue the counterattack with full intensity until the whistle blows.

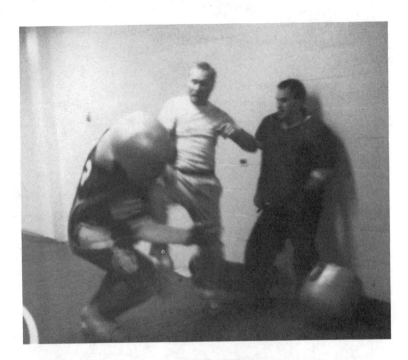

A kick to the groin has pitched the Bulletman's head forward. The fighter steps forward immediately for the knee to the head shot. This is a devastating blow, even more so when the knee to the head occurs when the Bulletman is getting himself up off the mat and his head is low.

It does not matter much what people think before stepping up to a scenario, because any such "thinking" occurs in their superconscious minds. The scenarios engage a whole other part of the brain that doesn't even know that superconscious part exists. This virtually never fails. The body doesn't know the difference and responds biochemically to the fight scenario simulation as if it was an actual attack.

When I face the Bulletman, see that predatory body carriage, feel the projection of his hostile intent, and then hear him shout something like, "Hey, shithead! What the fuck are you looking at?" at that point, I am partially transported mentally. My mind and body go immediately into that "Danger—relax and handle this properly or get

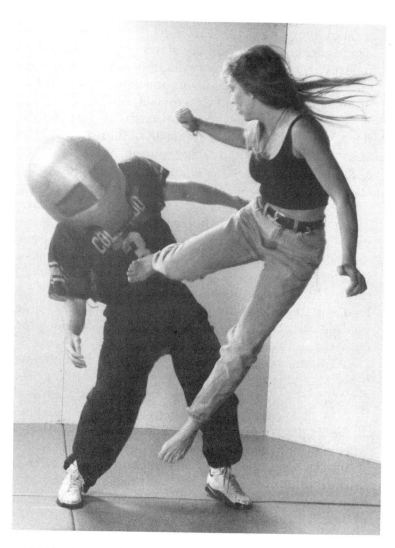

A bit flamboyant and not the first choice of technique for the street. But Kim, being a black belt, had to have a shot at the flying kick on the Bulletman. Besides, as I said, there are many kinds of beauty.

hurt bad" mode. After the fight, I often do not recall exactly what the Bulletman's attack was or what I did to defeat it. My loss of memory detail is one of the effects of adrenalization, and most everyone who does a fight scenario experiences it (more on this later).

From my personal experience during my bouncer days, I can tell you for a fact that all of these same adrenal stress effects occur both before, during, and after an actual fight. By way of further example, I recall another fight scenario when I was attacked by surprise from behind while I was teaching a class. The next thing I was aware of was being on top of the guy and giving out "karate yells" (*Kiyae*) as I pounded repeated and powerful overhead shutos to his neck. Then some part of my brain realized this guy was still conscious, and then, "How could this be?" passed through my mind. At that moment I realized something was in the way of my blows, and I began peeling back the helmet to get to the enemy's neck for a more damaging shot.

At about the same time, I realized that someone was blowing a whistle directly into my ear. At that point I returned to superconscious mind and realized, "Oh yeah, this is a class and . . . it's just a scenario." Even so, many of the residual physical effects of the adrenaline reaction were still with me (these include, among other things, enhanced alertness, speed and power, some fear, some time and memory distortion, and a basic "buzz and a half" for sure). That was fairly early in my experience with this training method, but even now, having done a number of the scenarios, I never fail to feel significant adrenal effects in most every scenario.

I repeat, some adrenal effects manifest themselves both before, during, and after the actual "fight."

Freezing Up

Adrenaline is a chemical that the body introduces into the bloodstream under the stress of what is perceived as a dangerous situation. It is sometimes called the fight-or-flight response. Most species experience this reaction. The adrenal response is particularly extreme under the stress of combat.

Since the fight scenarios engage this adrenal response, the fighter learns to use and control this biochemistry rather than letting it control him.

Some of you may have heard stories about people who, having been passengers in the front seat of a car during a crash, later tell how the driver inexplicably neither hit the brakes nor turned the wheel before their car crashed into another automobile (which was making the left turn, or whatever). The passenger explains that there seemed to be plenty of time to brake or turn, but the driver "just froze up!"

The driver's failure to brake or turn is a classic example of the effects of adrenal stress. This is combined with the "tachy psyche" effect on the passenger, which makes things appear to move in slow-motion. This effect experienced by the passenger is also a result of adrenalization and occurs not because the scene slows down, of course, but because the passenger's mind *speeds up* in its ability to process the visual cues of the life-threatening emergency. This is why people often report that things appeared to happen in slow-motion after a traumatic event.

The most advanced combat mind-set actually allows one to see everything as if it were happening in slow-motion while maintaining a relaxed mind that allows him to move and respond instantly and fluidly. This does not come together real often, but myself, Mike, and the Chinaman can report having experienced it. Therefore, I know it is possible.

We will get into this tachy psyche aspect more later on, but at this point let me say that conditioning oneself to use the survival-enhancing properties of the adrenaline reaction (as in perceiving that events are occurring more slowly) while deconditioning the negative effects (as in choking like a pig in a total freeze-up show) is as close to a martial arts "secret" as I have ever come across.

Let's consider another familiar example of freezing

up under stress. This one comes from that remarkable interface between the animal kingdom and man, namely, the two-lane blacktop—the highway. Perhaps you may have heard someone use an expression such as, "He was frozen stiff, I mean, like a deer frozen in the headlights." It is a fact that a deer will often freeze when crossing a road when it caught in the glare of oncoming car headlights. This is partly an adrenal reaction and partly because the deer's evolutionary survival strategies primarily involve either running or standing perfectly still in the hope that the predator won't notice it.

Unfortunately for the deer, the headlights are an unfamiliar stimulus, and so while the adrenal reaction is very high, at the same time the deer is denied any cues with which it is familiar and thus cannot determine which strategy is correct, flight or fight. Hence, it's a freeze-up job. The deer's freezing in the headlights is an example of the adrenal response preventing the use of muscles when they are needed most. It is not dramatically different with human beings.

If an individual has never faced stand-up aggression or violence before, then that individual will often freeze up and choke when confronted with it. As I related ad nauseam in my first book, the aggressor or bully is counting on this freeze-up or choke reaction on some level, and when he sees it he often attacks right then . . . and when he does not, he often gives up his plan to attack.

This is why it is essential to train in a way that gives the fighter the opportunity to learn to control these adrenal responses, and the only way this can be done is to first elicit them. Scenario training with the Bulletman makes this not only possible but actually predictable and reliable. The practical self-defense benefits of getting used to the adrenal reaction are enormous. I believe it is more important in a real fight than polished technical skill. There are many facets to this reality, which are all integrated into the same whole. Yet this training method has struck me from the very first as being a case where the whole is somehow greater than the sum of its parts.

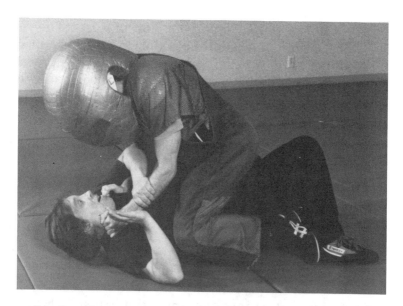

Sometimes the scenarios start out with everything having already gone wrong for the fighter. This fighter's face mirrors his initial shock, but in the next instant the adrenal stress itself will be the initiator for the escape technique. We already see the technique developing with the fighter's cross grab and heel of palm strike.

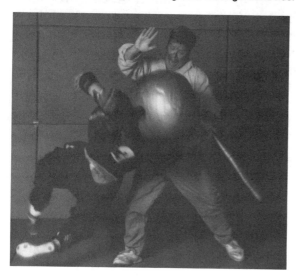

A good shot with the iron palm technique clearly knocks the Bulletman off his feet. Only a very large person would not be knocked down by this blow. Again, the Bulletman is not given a chance to fully chamber and get the stick moving before his weapon arm is trapped. Notice I have once again stepped past the assailant and maintain the "projection" of force after the blow has been struck. As Master Toyoda says, "Don't break it down," meaning make the movement fluid and complete by the use of follow-through. Do not interrupt the inertial flow.

Controlling and Timing the Flow of Adrenaline

Proper mind includes the ability to control and harness the positive effects of adrenal stress while suppressing the dysfunctional ones. This means recognizing the first precursor, the interview, and dealing with it effectively and immediately.

It is also important to realize that the mind-set needed to do this is also a very big part of the mind-set you need to have if it actually comes to an actual physical fight.

Once blows are struck (or to a somewhat less extent, once you decide a preemptive strike is required), the adrenaline will flow rather quickly into your bloodstream. But the positive adrenal effects of greater speed, power, tolerance to pain, and so on can come at the expense of higher brain functions.

Therefore, a person who "turns on full" during the start of an interview has impaired himself. He has impaired his higher cognitive brain functions, which are needed to deal with the interview properly, and he has limited his basic observational field as well (tunnel vision syndrome). Worse, the peak adrenal effect, where you experience superhuman strength, speed, power, and tolerance to pain, is fairly short-lived, and a quick burst at maximum intensity is all you get. You don't want to squander it before the physical fight begins. You want it to peak just when you need it, not before and not after. (Granted, one often feels the adrenal "buzz" for a long time during and after combat, but after the initial rush of adrenaline, it peaks quickly, and this is the point where its effects are most useful. During this stage one is very seldom even aware of the adrenaline buzz, because the peak adrenal state seldom involves the superconscious mind. It is only after you come down from this transitory peak state that you become consciously aware that you are still "buzzed out" on adrenaline.)

The person who adrenalizes too quickly must fight right then to be able to use it best, because after that first peak adrenal response, any second adrenal reaction is not nearly as powerful or useful. This too-quick adrenalization also manifests itself as the freeze-up reaction in someone who is not adrenal stress conditioned.

On the other hand, the person who is too slow to adrenalize may not get the full adrenal effect until he has already lost the fight or is impaired by injury.

I have seen more than a few such people who, being ambushed and knocked down (even hit or kicked a few times while on the ground), do not even start fighting until all that activity has sunk into their minds and been analyzed and then recognized for what it was.

As an odd example, I can recall three occasions where these slow-to-adrenalize people got up off the floor as their assailant was walking away (the assailant believing the fight was over and won) and then going Frankenstein as they went after their assailant, tearing him apart. My ex-bouncer pals report similar tales. But these are the exceptions that prove the rule. Adrenalizing too late can be as dysfunctional as adrenalizing too soon or choking.

DEVELOPING MUSCULAR MEMORY

The idea of developing muscular memory by learning to execute striking techniques full force under adrenal stress is a key to training people to defend themselves with this method. I will begin with some observations I made about myself some time after a particularly hairy knife attack I experienced (from which I still carry scars to this day). This fight was an extremely powerful adrenal experience.

I experienced auditory exclusion similar to what I experienced in the previously related fight scenario where the Bulletman attacked me by surprise and I failed to hear the whistle being blown directly in my ear for a while. In the actual barroom knife attack, because of the adrenal stress, I could not hear the other bar workers, including two big bouncers working with me, yelling at me at the top of their lungs, "He's done!" "He's finished!" Thus I continued to hold the knifer against the wall with one hand and repeatedly blasted him with my free right hand. After a while I realized the knifer had been unconscious for some time and I was the only thing holding him up. The guy's face was a raspberry jam job, and it took 32 stitches to sew my arm and hand back up. (He drew prison time for the attack, too—not, by the way, his first knife attack or his first prison term.)

My vision had definitely tunneled in on the knifer, and all the people calling out to me were standing no closer than about 15 feet away. This was because they could see I was "out of it," that is, in an adrenal state such that if they grabbed ahold of me, or even got too close, I might not be able to discriminate them from the enemy and might attack them on reflex.

Now for the point of all this. Having experienced the adrenal lesson of that particular knife attack, I was walking down the bar a few weeks later, and I saw this guy walking directly up to me at a brisk and determined pace. When his hand disappeared behind his back to reach for something in a quick motion, my body leaped over to the other side of the bar. Note that I say "my body leaped" over the bar, because the first moment my conscious mind was aware of anything out of the ordinary, I was already on the other side of the bar. To an extent, the little voice in my head asked, "What are we doing over here?"

The adrenal reaction of the knife fight had been processed, and a new reflex was now "in my body." It was the guy's hand reaching behind him suddenly (as it turned out, only to check to see if he still had his wallet before he left the bar) that triggered this new reflexive response.

Now, lest you think I'm a paranoid psycho, let me also relate that the guy was pissed off at his buddies over some sort of ribbing they were giving him, and he was storming out of the place. It was likely his quick, unplanned departure that made him check to see if he'd left his wallet behind. I misinterpreted his angry face and determined walk for potential hostility toward yours truly. My response was immediate because my conscious mind was never consulted.

When we train people under the adrenal stress of the fight scenarios, a similar type of learning occurs. Their subconscious minds are conditioned to respond to the woof as well as the attack on a different level of consciousness.

I will point out that the ability to develop this type of mind-set and to respond to an attack reflexively is often put forth as the ultimate goal of Asian systems of martial art when they are practiced for their self-defense value. It is referred to as *mushien*, or no mind. It must also be noted that very few persons studying martial art systems ever develop any such ability. In contrast, once the adrenal stress element is put into the equation (as in the fight scenarios), some level of this automatic-response phenomenon is always achieved.

Learning that Occurs Under Adrenal Stress is Stored in the Brain Differently and Occurs at an Accelerated Rate

My experience in observing students who have trained under adrenal stress suggests that such conditions have the effect of maximizing retention of learned skills. Consider this excerpt from the *New York Times* concerning research done at the Center for Neurobiology of Learning at the University of California at Irvine, James L. McGaugh, director:

> The "flight or fight" reaction has long been known to physiologists; the heart beats faster, the muscles are readied, and the body is primed in the most primitive of survival instincts. These and other distinctive reactions are triggered by the release into the bloodstream of the hormones adrenaline and noradrenaline.
>
> The same two hormones, it now appears, also prime the brain to take very special note in its memory banks of the circumstances that set off the flight or fight reaction.

The study goes on to make the following observation:

> ... suggests that the brain has two mem-
> ory systems, one for ordinary information
> and one for emotionally charged informa-
> tion. This emotional memory system has
> evolved because it had great survival value.

Could not have expressed it better myself. However, being academically oriented, the article says, "*had*" great survival value. There is no "had" about it; the only thing that has changed in modern society is that the adrenal reaction is suppressed, just as is the warrior spirit for the most part. This biochemistry is still there in everybody; it simply has to be exercised to be made more accessible to the individual in a crisis. (In women this drive expresses itself most obviously as the "maternal instinct" for pro-tection of the young. Mothers are legendary for their supernatural feats of strength and courage when defend-ing their children.) This is why scenario-based training is so demonstrably more effective than any other method. In fact, it can be argued that some level of exercising this warrior spirit, a communication with one's "animalistic self," is necessary to one's mental health. I see it as sim-ply getting in touch with one's "complete self."

Not only is learning that occurs under adrenal stress stored differently in the brain, but empirical evidence has made it clear to me that it is more efficient. That is, skills are learned much more rapidly under properly con-ducted adrenal conditioning exercises. This is what makes it possible for a weekend self-defense program to have such a dramatic effect in improving a person's real-world ability to either spot and thus avoid an attack or fight powerfully if need be. My confidence in making this assertion is based on the fact that these results are both demonstrative and repeatable.

Adrenal-Stress-Based Learning
Stays with the Individual Forever

There is another observation that I feel is significant about developing muscular memory under adrenal stress. Everybody involved in these adrenal stress conditioning programs has noted that individuals who take the basic course and then come back a year or so later (not having practiced at all in the interval) are invariably better when they return a year later than they were the final day of their original class. By "better" I mean that the power, accuracy, and timing of their strikes are better. Their handling of the woofing stage is also improved, as they are more relaxed and more decisive.

I attribute this phenomenon to the supposition that learning at the neurobiological level continues months (perhaps much longer) after the actual adrenal experience itself as the mind and body process the information and organize the neural networks necessary to execute a physical action (muscular memory) with an absolute minimum of processing by the cerebral cortex (conscious mind). Now, when this level of instantaneous response is combined with the ability to strike a living, moving assailant (as in the fight scenarios) with full power to the vulnerable targets of the body, then the fighter will very likely do just that in an actual encounter. In fact, in the absence of any previous conditioning (such as martial arts training), this is all the fighter knows how to do under such stress. You need to think about what that last statement means. I will provide a real world example.

There was a woman who took our basic course and then, about a year later, took another course in self-defense for women, sponsored by a group of police officers. Since they had some experience in the real world, the officers were using a "padded assailant" as an aide in teaching the women to hit. Unfortunately, the instructor chose our student to be the first one to make a knee strike to his groin. The officer was wearing commercially manufactured "armor" sometimes used in police training called a "Red Man" suit. Since we train our fighters to strike with full power, that is exactly what she did. The result was that the instructor was knocked unconscious by her first blow, and when he recovered he was unable to continue with the class.

Once a person has learned to execute a technique with full power under adrenal stress, adrenal stress itself is the cue that elicits that motor skill. Further, that motor skill tends to be executed in the same fashion as it was learned during the adrenal stress training episodes.

Consequently, since our student was likely a little nervous in front of the class and a bit stressed out by seeing the guy in the suit, *voila*—a beauty groin shot is born.

Also, the Red Man suit is simply not good enough to protect someone against a full-power shot from an adrenal-stress-trained individual (even when, as in this case, the woman striking the blow weighed less than 110 pounds and the officer receiving it weighed more than 200 pounds).

The armored assailant training method allows the fighter to learn how to strike the most powerful blow she can by direct feedback during adrenal stress. In other words, the fighter knows when the shot is good by the way it feels and by the reaction of the Bulletman. This action is then repeated and refined in each new scenario, and thus correct muscular memory begins to be established.

If there is a better way to teach people (actually, they teach themselves) how to hit real hard, I have yet to see it. The nature of learning under adrenal stress is at the root of why this method is so effective.

However, consider these factors as well. In a traditional martial arts dojo, dojang, or kwoon, the only full-contact striking that is done (if any) is on a heavy bag or air shield held by a training partner. I am not saying this type of exercise has no value; it does, and we use it ourselves. But hitting a static object like a heavy bag or air shield is useful only for getting the "static" mechanics of the blow, and this is often not enough to have any decent chance of landing the shot in a real fight. This is simply because there is much more to landing a solid shot on a real person in a real fight than simply the static mechanics of it.

WHY TRADITIONAL MARTIAL ARTS TRAINING IS INCOMPLETE PREPARATION FOR AN ACTUAL SELF-DEFENSE ENCOUNTER

I guess I could write a book on this topic, and in fact I have, but once again I will not try your patience with a rehash of that.

At this point you should have the idea that it is all the stuff that precedes the actual throwing of the first blow in a fight that often decides the outcome of the actual physical battle, and that it is the way you handle this stuff (the interview and woof, and so on) that will often determine whether there will be a fight at all.

As Musashi said it several centuries ago, "The battle is decided before first swords are crossed."

Now, you can read Musashi's words with the adolescent mind that wants (needs) to believe that there are mystic secrets in such sayings, or you can simply see

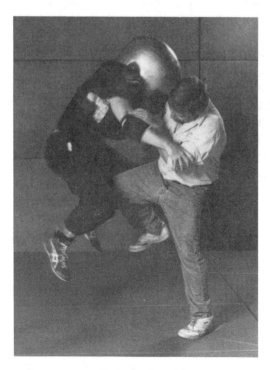

This knee strike to the groin has knocked the Bulletman off his feet on impact. It is difficult to learn how to do this without actually being able to deliver a full-force knee to a person's groin. The armor makes this possible, and people learn the technique pretty quickly. Notice I have turned my head to the side. This is because when a person is struck this hard in the groin, his head will always slam forward and could hit you in the face with enough force to knock you out.

them as what they are: observations (always imperfectly translated) by people who have had some experience with battle and, having reflected on the experience, communicated their impressions and/or analysis of same. Indeed, we are lucky to get this, because most times what we get are second- or third-hand reports from people who weren't there and didn't have to fight.

The classical Asian method of martial arts training does not address any of the elements of the interview and does not involve any scenario-type training. Thus, the enormously important element of actual, real-world self-defense is not addressed at all. The student of a classical Asian system may not be aware that they exist, much less understand their significance. Without an understanding of the interview and the woof, and in the absence of adrenal stress conditioning, the martial arts student's first real fight can be quite a sudden-impact learning experience.

For the most part, Asian systems concentrate on technique, that is, the physical "how to do it" part. But since the reality of how actual fights occur is absent from the traditional martial arts training model, many of the techniques taught in martial arts classes are not only useless in a real fight, they are actually dangerous. Well, maybe I shouldn't sugar-coat it like this . . . because actually, once the fists start flying, things can go from bad to much worse for the fighter trained only in an Asian martial system.

The classical Asian training method concentrates on developing fine motor skills in the execution of technique. But fine motor skills are the first thing to go under adrenal stress. Hence, even when we narrow our focus to the handful of basic, real-world-relevant techniques that are taught in classical Asian martial systems, martial arts students may find even these techniques unavailable to them because under adrenal stress they cannot perform them. Now, read this paragraph again.

On more than a few occasions I have found myself among a group of martial arts instructors debating the topic, "Does martial arts study help or hinder most people in a real fight?" The consensus most often comes down to the recognition that, for most people, martial arts study does not help them, but for a few, martial arts training makes all the difference in the world. (Keep in mind I am limiting this "consensus" to martial arts instructors who have actually done some real street fighting and therefore are in a position to have an informed and educated opinion on the subject.)

Some of these instructors will say this is because most people do not stay at their martial arts training long enough to develop the skill level necessary to prevail in a real fight. Personally, I must reject this explanation and might counter that perhaps one is only able to fight after years of studying the martial system because it takes that long to overcome the handicaps of the systems techniques and training method. But that would be to digress into a secondary issue.

The way I see it, teaching self-defense by the traditional Asian method for most people is like teaching someone how to swim without ever putting them in the water.

Imagine that you are given the task of teaching a group of people to swim who have never been in the water before. To add interest to your work, after you provide the group with your instructional method, they will all be taken out for the Big Boat Ride. And yes, you guessed correctly, after they get about a mile off shore, they will all be tossed out of the boat and abandoned. The effectiveness of your training method will be determined by the number of survivors.

Now, consider that we add these additional elements to our imaginary scenario. On top of the fact that your entire family and wife or girlfriend are in the class, you are given a critical choice: either you can have two years to train the swim class (before the Big Boat Ride test), or you can train them in only one weekend. If you choose the two-year deal, you can try anything you want to get them ready in that time, but you cannot actually use any water in your training. But if you go for the short weekend training period, you can have the use of a big swimming pool.

Traditional martial arts can be seen as being like the case where the instructor takes the two-year, no-actual-water-training approach. Perhaps you can visualize this: all the students in swim trunks (instead of karate gis), moving their arms in swimming motions, all in unison, of course. Later in this "no water" swimming program, the students actually lie on the wooden floor on their bellies while moving their arms and kicking their legs in swimming motions. After only four or five months of this, the students have developed real endurance. They have stamina and are in good physical condition. They can even look good at what they are doing, especially when they are training in a large group.

If they are lucky they might get a pep talk from a swimmer who has actually been in the water before. It might sound like this: "Okay, people, remember, when that water hits you, it's going to be cold, and you might have trouble breathing for an instant, but just keep kicking those legs and throwing those arms into the water and, most of all, swimmers, *relax* and flow, don't fight the water, relax and swim people . . . SWIM!"

Actually, it's not bad advice, but how many of the class will have the contextual framework required to benefit from hearing it (having never been in the water before)? The morning after the Big Boat Ride, how many fewer people in that class will not be found washed up on the beach, belly-up, because of that inspirational pep talk?

Now, consider the alternative case where the instructor goes for the one-weekend training period with a swimming pool at his disposal. How much time would be spent on teaching "swimming technique," that is, showing the people how to move their arms and legs when they actually get into the water?

If the instructor were doing the job correctly, very little time would be spent on the academics of swimming technique, and even less or none on proper swimming form. The students would just be pushed off the diving board into the deep end of the pool and allowed to splash around a bit until they learned to tread water. Slower learners would be rescued when they began to go under for the second or third time. Then, after a reasonable rest period they would be given a few pointers and then thrown back in the pool until they discovered how to tread water for a little while. Next they would be given a demonstration of how to go from a treading water position to a swimming position. Then they would return to the pool to try it themselves. The objective would be to give them as much water time as was possible without exhausting them such that the recovery periods became counterproductive or they risked being defeated in spirit.

I submit that after the first day, most of the class would already be swimming at some level and could teach themselves the rest just by staying in the pool. This would leave the instructor time for individual help and tune-ups for the students who really needed it.

Now, I ask you, which group do you think would have the most faces in the post-Big Boat Ride graduation picture? The wooden-floor, no-water boys who studied for years . . . or the weekend swimming pool class?

It is as easy to understand why so many more people would avoid drowning in the weekend class as it is to see why the two-year no-water boys would have such high casualties.

What is more difficult for some people to appreciate is that this analogy can be carried over fairly directly to self-defense training. Throwing the fighter into the "fight scenario" is the equivalent of throwing the swimming student into that swimming pool. It puts learning on a very accelerated track because it engages powerful survival instincts.

Now, not having been overly charitable in my description of the effectiveness of the traditional Asian systems in teaching real-world self-defense, let me relate a tale that shows the other side of the coin. Namely, "The Asimo Man and His Lake Tahoe Tae Kwon Do Killers."

The average class in our Colorado training program generally has three or four ranking black belts out of the usual 15 attendees, though no previous martial arts training is required.

One year, one of these black belts was Asimo, a TKD instructor and third-degree black belt who had a dojang near Lake Tahoe, California. After taking our five-day program, Asimo asked us to come to his dojang in California to put on a weekend version of the training. (We had developed the weekend program in response to the fact that coming all the way to Colorado for five days was too expensive for many people.)

Asimo is an individual with a rare, adventurous spirit, and his students were very well-disciplined. When we taught the class at his dojang, his students did very well. However, the first time we taught the course to them, Asimo's students and instructors had most of the same problems as all martial arts people do in their first few fight scenarios. In particular, karate or TKD people will often (as a result of previous training, and sparring in particular) attempt techniques that are not appropriate or safe to try in a real fight. Hence, these techniques are not rewarded in the fight scenarios. For example, if the fighter throws a roundhouse kick to the Bulletman's head, the Bulletman just grabs his leg or tackles him and takes him to the ground. If the fighter throws a slight point-type technique, the Bulletman ignores it and takes the fighter to the ground or otherwise frustrates the movement. The Bulletman only responds to well-placed, solid shots, primarily knock-out shots.

At first, since martial arts people generally have never actually hit anyone with full power, their chamber of depth is off, and they are either too close or too far away when they strike. This means the shot has little knock-down potential when it arrives. The more common error is throwing the shot from too far away rather than too close. I suppose it may be true that many martial arts people have more difficulty in their first few fight simulations than a lot of untrained people in the class.

Now, let's return to the specific case of our Lake Tahoe TKD Killers.

By the end of the first weekend training period, Asimo's tae kwon do boys were connecting pretty good.

They were sticking to the basic power techniques and had abandoned any attempts at fancy Hollywood spin kicks and such. Some were connecting with real good power, and fairly regularly. They had significantly overcome any initial denial or fear reaction to the woof and were clearly better able to maintain their composure and motor control.

Still, though it was a very good class, even one of our better-performing classes, the first year at Lake Tahoe was nothing compared to the second year, when we came back for a repeat performance of the basic class and had most of the same people. Once again, we saw the phenomenon of a group that comes back after a year and is dramatically better than it was at the conclusion of its first basic class.

In the case of the Lake Tahoe TKD Killers, I attribute the significant amplification of this often-observed effect to their muscular memory interfacing with their years of emphasis on proper body mechanics in their study of TKD's power-striking techniques. But, after the first basic class, they had the other parts of the puzzle—those involving the maintenance of motor control under adrenal stress. In addition, the basic class experience had calibrated their power shots (range-, entrance-, and timing-wise) for striking on a moving, living aggressor. This includes the idea of chamber of depth, footwork, and all the rest.

The result was that the second year we were in Lake Tahoe, these guys hit so hard that it was, for the first time really, pressing the limits of the body armor technology as well as the skill of the some of the best Bulletmen who ever put on armor.

When I saw them hit the Bulletmen in the head with their hands or elbows, the Bulletmen's feet just snapped out from under them. I was confident that some of those blows would actually be fatal if delivered on a human being not protected by the armor of the helmet and shoulder pad anchoring system we use. It was a real horror show for sure for the Bulletmen. The incident of the Lake Tahoe Killers has now become a legend in Bulletman folklore.

At the conclusion of that second class, I basically told these guys that there was nothing more they really needed to learn about how to hit hard. I also remember pointing out that their blows could be crippling or fatal and cautioning them to recognize this and use them with discretion.

This case is a prime example of the other side of the coin—the value of traditional martial training in imparting the proper body mechanics of striking a powerful blow. But it is also an example that highlights the shortcomings of the traditional Asian method because of their lack of scenario training. Traditional martial arts training simply does not provide an opportunity for full-contact striking on a living, moving, woofing assailant in an authentic fight simulation.

CHAPTER FIVE

Toward a More Realistic View of Asian Martial Systems

While many will argue otherwise, I submit that if you are diligent and truly objective in researching the historical record of the Asian founding masters, it becomes clear that their intention was to establish an *art*, not a fighting system for real-world self-defense. Self-defense was not their interest; after all, most of those founding masters had never been in a real fight either.

While there is certainly applied self-defense value to be found in classical systems and their techniques, the individual will never realize that value simply by "learning" to perform those techniques in the dojo.

CLASSICAL MARTIAL ARTS AS "ANCIENT AND PROVEN COMBAT SYSTEMS"

For about a decade and a half, there has been a heated ongoing debate in such magazines as *Black Belt*. Periodically, letters to the editor will comment on the previous month's article, which had a title such as "Boxing vs. Karate." (This is a subject that has been written and rewritten to death by these type magazines in one form or another for more than two decades.) Without fail, some reader will write something like the following:

> It is absurd to compare boxing to karate! Boxing is a sport and karate is a self-defense system designed for real-world, life-and-death combat. Karate is the result of more than a thousand years of development, and its techniques are the ones that have survived and proven themselves on the battlefield.

This is a colorful description of karate for sure, but it is factually incorrect in every detail. For the most part, it would not be a valid description of any other weaponless fighting system or art either. Consider the following.

1) *Karate as practiced in the dojo is a sport.*

Karate as practiced in the dojo is not a self-defense system; it is a sport. It precisely represents what a sport is supposed to be—that is, a game with rules whereby participants can demonstrate their skill against their opponents in a safe and controlled manner such that the potential for serious injury is reduced to a very low level.

In most karate schools, no contact is allowed at all at the lower belts, and even at black belt level, there is seldom any real, full-power contact, especially to the head.

Contrast this with boxing, which, while also a sport, is much more like a real fight than anything one will ever likely see in a karate dojo. Boxing is full-contact, full-power mostly all the time. Blood is spilled regularly in boxing. In a boxing match, you demonstrate your ability by slugging it out in the ring with a guy who's determined to take your head off. Knockouts are fairly common, and they always decide the victor when they do occur.

On the other hand, an actual knockout in a karate competition most often represents an "accident" and will generally disqualify the person who delivered the blow, thus making his opponent lying on the canvas the "victor."

It is nearly impossible to achieve any level of success in boxing without developing the psychological preparedness to engage the enemy. Contrast this with karate (in its many forms), where there are many black belts, even instructors, who do not even have an acquaintance with the very concept of proper psychological preparedness to engage the enemy. After years of karate training, they may never have been really hit in their lives (even in the dojo by accident!). Nor have they ever really hit anybody else.

Yet somehow, by what magic escapes me, they are expected to do it all right somehow, the first time out, in defending themselves against a real-world attack.

These are the facts. Now, which sounds more like a sport to you, boxing or karate? At first glance, which seems like the better preparation for a street fight?

(2) *Karate has never been proven in combat, since no war has ever been fought using karate, nor any other unarmed martial art for that matter.*

Can you imagine the following scene? A few hundred guys on one side of the battlefield raise their naked fists and cut loose with martial arts cries, while on the other side of the battlefield, a few hundred other guys do the same. Next, the two forces clash and decide the outcome with fists, feet, and throws.

It has never happened, people, and it is not likely that it ever will. Weapons have been the first choice in both war and individual combat since prehistoric times.

The Uncommon Quality of Common Sense

Of course, all this is no more than common sense, but if you present these obvious historical facts to some dedicated martial artist, you will soon discover how uncom-

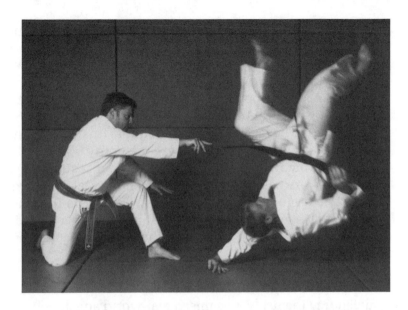

The main application of this type of throw is for publication on the covers of martial arts magazines. I have never used a throw like this in an actual fight. However, the principles and concepts that performing these types of techniques explore are involved in every real-world type throw. Again, note the follow-through and projection of intent in this throw. Actually, my performance of this aikido technique is pretty sloppy. But since most people have not learned to take falls, being thrown like this (particularly into a fire hydrant or parked car) could do some real damage. (Especially if it was Mike Haynack or Robert Stein doing the throwing, because they actually know some aikido.)

mon a thing common sense really is. People will believe principally what they wish to believe, which is another way of saying what they feel they need to believe.

Many martial artists will feel compelled to offer counter examples of specific historical fights (often by the founding master of their art) that demonstrate the combat effectiveness of their system.

In reality, such incidents, when they actually occurred at all, only tested and demonstrated that specific individual's ability at that specific time and in that specific type of conflict.

Who is doing the fighting is always more important

than the particular art or style being employed. (While I am pontificating on this, let me add that who is doing the instructing is often more important than the particular art being taught. As my pal the Eagle is fond of saying, "the students always reflect the instructor.")

Finally, how about this "thousand-year-old heritage" idea?

Tae kwon do (TKD), the most practiced form of karate in the world as it is practiced today, was really "invented" in the 1950s by Korean General Choi Hong Hi. The general had an opportunity to see Japanese karate training during the almost two decades of military occupation of his country by a brutal Japanese military force. Seeing the Japanese practice recreational kendo and karate, he wanted the Korean people to have a form of their own to practice as an expression of their own culture.

When the Japanese occupation ended after World War II, the general created tae kwon do as an expression and symbol of Korean national unity. The encouragement of a nationalistic spirit in Korea, after the humiliating years of military occupation, was correctly seen by the general as essential to rebuilding his country.

However, to achieve this, the general wanted to make sure that the new Korean art was not confused with the foreign occupiers' karate. General Choi wanted everyone to know immediately when they saw a TKD exhibition that it was not the Japanese karate. This is why he added the high and fancy kicking techniques for which TKD is known. They were never intended as combat techniques.

TKD is taught to all members of the Republic of Korea (ROK) armed forces. But this is really for the same reason pugil stick training and calisthenics are practiced by most armies of the world—namely, to develop combat spirit and as a physical exercise to keep the troops in a state of good physical conditioning.

The techniques of TKD, for the most part, were never based on any actual hand-to-hand combat experience by anyone, nor were they truly designed for actual hand-to-hand fighting. The ROK trooper is generally quite dedicated and tough, but he is not expected to take on an invasion by North Korean Communists empty-handed with tae kwon do.

So what about Japanese karate? Karate was unheard of in Japan until about the 1930s. The real motivation for the development of Japanese martial arts as we know them today appears to have been an effort on the part of specific individuals (most of whom lived in this century) to maintain a martial tradition after the samurai warrior class had been dissolved. These individuals could often trace their warrior class heritages back for many generations.

When the warrior class, trained in the use of the sword, bow, and spear, were no longer needed, these individuals wished to keep the traditions of such martial service alive by turning their practice into an art that could be enjoyed by all. In order to do this, the warrior arts had to be made safer to practice. The development of the sport of judo by Master Kano from the jujutsu and aki-jutsu is an example of this. Fundamentally, this is how all the various Japanese karate styles developed.

The founder of aikido, O' Sensei (Great Teacher), Morihei Ueshiba only died in 1969. Sort of tough to get a thousand-year history out of all that for today's martial arts, isn't it?

Some will be quick to say, "Yeah, but it was all based on Chinese kung fu, which is a thousand years old or more." Once again, people will believe what they want or what they feel they need to believe.

"Kung fu" is actually a term invented by Americans (just like "Peking" for "Beijing") to describe scores of individual weapons arts simply called "wu shu," or "war arts" by the Chinese. Kung fu can be translated from Chinese to mean simply "to work hard" or "to practice hard."

The traditions of kung fu as we see them today seem to have begun a little more than a century and a half ago, principally by Shaolin monks. Most of these were spear and Chinese broadsword arts, even though now we tend to think of kung fu as being principally an unarmed form of fighting. (By the way, when the political climate went sour on them, those Shaolin monks were all slaughtered in their own temples by soldiers with swords and spears, and very quickly at that.)

Please understand, I am not saying these martial arts have no self-defense value; they often do. What I am calling for is a more realistic understanding of how they actually developed and the difference between martial art study and applied self-defense study.

Now some might say, "What about the 'true masters'? Don't these people demonstrate the clear and undeniable self-defense value of their art?"

ARE THERE REALLY "TRUE MASTERS"?

If by using the term "true master," one means an individual who cannot be defeated in combat, then there are no true masters. Any man can be beaten; any man can be killed.

But in reflecting over some two and a half decades of my informal search for masters, there is a handful of persons whom I recognize as true masters of their art.

An example would be Fumio Demura-San, who got his paws on me back in 1972. Using his classical Japanese karate alone, he could almost certainly kill me in a real combat. Another would be judo Master Yoshisada Yonezuka-San. "Yoni" could throw anybody, anytime, anywhere, and amazingly hard. If it were an actual combat and Yoni had to throw someone (such as in defense of his family from a real attack), it would likely occur on concrete or on some other hard surface, not on a judo mat. The result of such a throw could be terminal. In any case, the assailant would certainly have multiple fractures and would not be capable of any further hostile action.

Toyoda-San, as I mentioned earlier, is an aikido master who learned his art from its founder Ueshiba, referred to as "O-sensei," as a youngster in Japan. O-sensei sent Toyoda to teach aikido in the United States. Although Toyoda did not speak English at that time and had virtually no money, he packed his bags and left for America (that warrior spirit, people). While some people in the aikido community call Toyoda's art "Chicago-style aikido," personally, I prefer to call it the "John Deere" school of aikido, because if Master Toyoda actually used his skills for combat effect against real assailants, those assailants (when being examined later in the city morgue) would likely be judged to have been killed in some sort of farm-machinery accident.

The inshin karate system founder, Shihan Joko Ninomiya, in Denver, is another karate master who would be a horror show plus to anyone foolish enough to try to attack him. His evasion of the blows and his footwork slip him to his attacker's blind side, where he is free to strike any blow, and I think even one strike from this guy would knock almost anyone unconscious or worse. He is one of the few people I have seen who can get neck snapping (lethal power) into a high roundhouse kick to the opponent's head.

Paul de Thouars is another martial artist I'd call a master. He is a master of the Indonesian art of penjat silat and founder of the bunta negra fighting system. This man has had to use lethal force in actual combat with the kris, an Indonesian style of fighting knife. (I noticed the knife scar on his leg and eventually wormed the tale out of him.) Though the pandekar, Paul de Thouars, is well past 60 years of age, any small group of thugs who tried to roll this "old man" would be in for a real horror show as well. The "Detour Man" (as he is sometimes fondly referred to) could hit you at will, and every time he did you'd see a different color and pattern of stars—that is, if you were still conscious enough to see those stars, which you wouldn't be, because most of his strikes are nerve-strike knock-out techniques. Paul de Thouars is one of the very few "nerve strike" artists I have dealt with who struck me as being able to make multiple nerve strike attacks work in real combat. These techniques are sometimes referred to as "light-force knockouts." (Even some people holding themselves out as "experts" in this area could have real problems making their light-force knockouts work on anyone other than a sitting-duck volunteer from a seminar audience.)

WHAT MAKES A MASTER?

First, allow me to point out the common characteristics of all the people I have had experience with and would term "masters."

1) Almost without exception they were born in the country of origin of the art they practice.

2) They began study of the art at a very early age, like 12 years old or younger.

3) They adopted the study and instruction of the art as their profession at an early age and continued in that activity as their sole profession throughout their adult life.

4) They have a good sense of humor combined with an indifferent attitude toward using lethal force if it should be necessary. In other words, while not "crazed killers," they would not hesitate to kill if required.

5) Their body types are particularly suited to the particular art they practice. (This is often a result of item number 1 above.)

6) These individuals have an obvious talent for the art. They have a natural facility for it, like some people have a talent for playing a musical instrument.

Now I ask you, what is the significance of these items? Well, *numero uno* is the fact that you can't duplicate these conditions for becoming a master in any training program. But there is another significant observation to be made here. Read item number 3 again.

The road to becoming a master of the art involves 20 or 30 years or more of applying techniques on students as well as on other masters. You can only do this if teaching the art is your profession for many years.

Consequently, combined with his natural talent for the art, the master has built up a tremendous amount of muscular memory, and thus all his art's techniques are fluidly accessible to him. It's all in his body, and his conscious mind need not be consulted.

Further, over the years he has dealt with virtually every kind of body type existent. The adaptation of both technique and tactics to different body structures is always a factor in a real battle. In applying nerve strikes, this is practically at the heart of the art. The master plays his assailant's body like a musical instrument. To do this, you first need to have a talent for music (percussion is a popular theme with masters). Given natural talent and then years of study with the instrument, one can actualize and develop talent, be it musical or martial. The master has both of these things, first the talent and then years of daily study to develop it. No training program can provide people with talent they don't have. It can only hope to actualize that which they do have. Fortunately, courtesy of the natural selection process, everyone has the animal instinct to survive (though a person may be somewhat out of touch with it temporarily due to a lack of adrenal experience).

Consequently, while I contend that it is impossible to train successfully to be a master, it is also my feeling that you need not be a master to have a good chance of avoiding or prevailing in a street battle.

Consider what this means concerning emulation of the master as a training strategy. Do you see that for most of us, to take this training strategy too far can be counterproductive? We are not the master; we can only learn from the master and adapt that knowledge to our own talents, body type, spirit, and so on, where applicable and possible for us. Perhaps this is a part of what Bruce Lee meant when he said, "Absorb what is useful."

VERY FEW REAL FIGHTS ARE DECIDED BY SUBTLE OR MASTER TECHNIQUE

Once again, real fights are almost always sloppy affairs. They seldom offer any display of formal martial training by either combatant. In my observation, this seems to be true regardless of whether the fighters are black belts or have no training at all. Hence, we arrive at the primary point of this book from another angle.

Let's review the central assertions put forth thus far, as follows:

1) The ability to control adrenal stress, rather than knowledge or skill at martial technique, is the central determining factor in how a person will really function in an actual attack

2) It is only by virtue of some level of adrenal stress conditioning that the mental state and motor control required to execute techniques can even exist (when it comes to a real fight, that is). Otherwise, people can simply choke and have no access to their knowledge of technique.

3) Adrenal conditioning requires an adrenal-eliciting experience. Any physical motor responses (techniques) learned under adrenalization become internalized through muscular memory. Thus, the technique cannot be "forgotten" under the stress of an attack. To the contrary, it is the adrenal stress of an attack that elicits the motor response. Without the adrenal stress element, any training in technique is simply incomplete for self-defense use.

4) The best way to learn to do technique in a proper

manner is to actually execute it full force on a real person, just as you would in an actual fight. When we train to hit a person with a powerful and disabling blow without ever actually hitting a person in our training, then we cannot really learn how to strike such a blow to our full potential. Nor can we develop the essential assured confidence in our hitting power.

5) The typical assailant is a bully at heart and often is only prepared for a victim, not an actual fight where he might be injured. Consequently, he employs the interview, and hence our opportunity to effect successful avoidance strategy by recognizing and handling the interview properly. Doing this demands maintaining some level of relaxation and calm under the visceral stress of stand-up aggression (the woof). If we have no experience with this woofing in our training, we are likely to be critically unprepared for same in an actual encounter.

6) While a master can make any style or technique work in combat, this is not truly relevant to training "regular" people to survive a real attack. We don't need to become masters to defend ourselves, nor is it likely that we could become masters anyway. Fancy technique is not needed in a real fight, and we do not need a whole lot of different techniques, either. What we need in a real fight is basic technique—gross motor skills that can be executed under stress and that contact with enough power on the correct targets to incapacitate our enemy.

The scenario-based training method addresses all of the above realities. It is not designed to turn out masters of technique. It is not designed to turn out people who look pretty while training or fighting. Neither does it assume that the student has any significant natural talent for fighting or will continue to study the system for years in order to develop self-defense competence in same.

WHAT THE SCENARIO TRAINING METHOD ACHIEVES

This adrenal-stress-based scenario training method is designed to increase a person's real-world self-defense and fighting ability by at least 100 percent—and do it in the space of a five-day course or even a weekend training program. I would not tell you that I believe that this program achieves this objective (virtually every time and with everybody) if I had not actually observed this reality by first-hand observation over several years.

Some of the people who take this course are advanced black belts (and better than I ever was at martial arts technique). Others who take the course have no previous self-defense or martial arts training of any kind.

It just doesn't matter. Regardless of where they start out, they improve their fighting ability—and their awareness and avoidance skills—dramatically through this training method.

Pretty bold statements, huh?

Keep in mind that, in an important sense, the scenario training method simply provides the opportune conditions under which people are able to discover and exercise their own natural (though repressed) survival instincts. It is precisely because everybody has this survival drive that the program works.

I am not claiming that this training method turns everybody into some kind of invincible fighter. That would be absurd, and besides, as I have noted already, *anyone can be beaten; anyone can be killed.* But I stand by the statement that this method improves everyone's self-defense and fighting ability very significantly.

Scenario Training Works for both
Black Belts and Untrained Fighters

Allow me to cite two examples of course attendees who were at opposite ends of the training and attitude spectrum: one, a black belt with some street fighting experience; the other, a woman with no previous training at all and, frankly, rather meek in her manner.

In a weekend course I observed that the woman was not making contact with her training partner in an angle of attack drill. The drill was simply a rehearsal of the path of a properly executed shuto strike to the opponent's carotid artery. The training partner (not the armored assailants) would simply reach to grab the student, and the student redirected the grab, trapped the arm, and in slow-motion executed the knife-hand strike, ending up with the edge of her hand on the training partner's neck, specifically on the carotid artery.

It was apparent to me that the woman was uncomfortable with the idea of even touching someone in what was a rehearsal for an act of violence. Hence, she did not actually touch the guy's neck. I had to work with her just to get her to start making even this level of physical contact. But I did not spend a lot of time on this because we had not had our first fight scenario yet, and I knew she had to have that adrenal experience before any of these mechanics of striking a blow would have any real meaning for her.

To cut to the chase, by the last day of the weekend course, this woman had broken her arm in one of the fight scenarios. (Occasionally, people will break bones in the fight scenarios. But let me say that it does not happen very often, and it occurs with even less frequency each new year we instruct the programs.) However, after going to the hospital and having the arm set and put in a cast, she returned to the course and basically demanded to have her final fight scenario! Having had a taste of her own inner strength, she wasn't going to let anything stop her. In this case, I had to respect her courage. So we taped her cast to her body and sent her in. It was a "portal of safety" scenario and the Bulletman came up, blocked her way and said, "Hey baby, nice tits, I think we should get together honey." Then he reached out for her. She brushed past this grab and in a determined voice commanded, "Keep your hands off of me!"

The Bulletman spun back directly in front of her and said, "Where do you think you're going now, sweetie?" Her response was a loud, "Right through you!" as she executed a perfect knee to the groin that lifted the Bulletman off his feet, followed by a second knee strike to the head as he recovered and his head pitched forward.

This shot would have knocked almost anyone unconscious—sweet contact with plenty of juice and virtually no telegraphing. This action represented a real breakthrough in this woman's conceptualization of what she was capable of doing. Once she began to make contact with her survival instincts in the first few fight scenarios and had experienced a portion of her own power, she would not even allow a broken arm to stop her from completing her journey.

Watching people make this transition is one of the real payoffs in teaching these classes, because it's all right there in front of you, and you can watch them stepping up and doing it.

Now let's consider our other example. This guy was a second-degree black belt, had done some bouncing, and had been in some street fights. In the first few fight scenarios he did well, better than average for sure, but I could see that he was experiencing elements of delayed stress in the fight simulations. He was in an altered state of consciousness in the scenarios, and his mind sped up ahead of his body under this adrenal stress.

This guy was landing some good shots right off the bat that would, in all probability, end the fight in the opening seconds. But he was a bit too "pumped up," such that he threw more shots than actually connected well and was using up his energy extremely quickly. This is what I mean by "his mind sped up ahead of his body."

Like I said, this guy could fight from day one; we didn't have to show him much along those lines. What he developed through the course was the ability to control his adrenal response such that he could relax more under the stress and use much less energy in the fights. If this guy had to fight more than one person at a time, this could make all the difference because he wouldn't burn out so fast.

The scenarios also tuned up the power transmission of his shots, because he was actually hitting something again. A slight difference in the step and perception of the chamber of depth in striking a blow can make the difference between a stunning shot and a flat knockout.

Perhaps most importantly, he developed the ability to let the woof go through him and not let his enemy control him by forcing him immediately into "attack-kill mode" with words alone. His tendency had been to adrenalize too quickly.

Once he got through the first three simulations, he was beginning to relax more, breathe properly, and use deescalation and avoidance strategies. Before he experienced the scenarios, I don't think he really would have been capable of doing this kind of deescalation and successfully applying an avoidance strategy. I'll say it again—a fight avoided is a fight won, because any fight has the potential for homicide, and that homicide could be yours no matter how good a fighter you are.

I would submit that both of these individuals—the 105-pound woman with no previous experience and a meek attitude at first and the black belt bouncer with some street fights under his belt—improved their real-world self-defense ability very significantly through this scenario-based training program.

The Scenarios Improve and Help Maintain My Own Fighting Skills

I try to do a fight scenario myself in each class, although since I'm instructing, I sometimes "worm out." The scenarios are stressful, and there is always a scary and unpleasant element to it. It is an adrenal event like sky diving—it can be fun, but there is always that element of primal fear at work.

But I always feel better after I step up and do one. Since I have not bounced in those bars for a lot of years, it brings me back to what a fight is really like—a little tunnel vision, some auditory exclusion, a burst of power and speed in the execution of a blow that under normal circumstances of training (like hitting the heavy bag) I cannot really duplicate. Just having the Bulletman woofing on me brings me back to a combat consciousness of absolute attention on the task at hand. The scenarios also help me to maintain survival habits like glancing about for a second assailant when one Bulletman is woofing on me to distract my attention from an attack from the rear by his companion.

CHAPTER SIX

Scenario-Based Training with Weapons

Weapons have always been the first choice for combat, and the modern personal weapons are the gun, the knife, and the stick. It behooves you to develop a familiarity with these weapons if you are serious about self-defense.

At the heart of self-defense is the greater concept of self-reliance. The brutal fact is that you cannot rely on anyone but yourself to protect you against being beaten, raped, or killed. The U.S. Supreme Court has even ruled quite explicitly that the police have no obligation to protect any individual from crime. They have only the general responsibility to "police" the community. As a simple matter of practicality, if you are attacked in the street, in your home, or anywhere else, most likely the only person who will be there to help you is *you!* Okay, this is pretty obvious, but over the years I have observed that fewer people than you might think have really accepted this reality.

Avoidance (which depends on awareness) is your first and best self-defense strategy, but once it comes to a fight, the weapon is always preferable to the empty hand. A weapon, such as a gun or knife, can allow you to defeat a physically larger and stronger enemy and even multiple assailants.

However, *proper combat mind-set is still the first requirement for effective self-defense*, whether you have a weapon or not. It is for this reason that we require people to take the basic empty-handed self-defense course before they can go on to any weapons course with us.

Because we are instructing applied self-defense for the real world and not martial arts, we have undertaken the teaching of the use of weapons. In doing so, we have adapted the principles of adrenal-stress-based scenario training to the use of weapons.

A PISTOL YOU DON'T HAVE WITH YOU WON'T HELP

First off, despite my criticism of the shortcomings of the martial arts training method for real-world self defense (which principally arise from its lack of adrenal stress scenario training), I know that martial arts training can have real-world self-defense value. Therefore, I stand in fundamental disagreement with those people who take the position, "Screw that kung fu shit—it won't work in a real fight, and besides, if anybody really fucks with me, I'll just shoot him."

When I hear this type of talk, most often it strikes me as coming from the banks of that age-old river in Egypt, namely, "de-nial!" People taking this macho-sounding "I'll just shoot them" position many times have not really accepted the possibility that at some time they may actually have to defend themselves effectively in order to have a chance of survival. Despite their bravado, they are basically in denial of the fact that such a situation could really happen to them and that they could be killed. They have not realistically visualized how an actual assault might happen to them. If they had, it would be much more difficult for them to hold onto this fantasy solution to their fear of being assaulted. Let's consider some facts.

First, consider the fact that most of the people who are doing all this talking about shooting people rarely have a gun on them when they make this little declaration.

Mike "the Amazing Eagle" Haynack once told me about spectators at self-defense demonstrations who would sometimes point their fingers at him as if pointing a gun and then, moving their thumbs like pistol hammers, pretend to shoot him. This action was an expression of their attitude toward martial arts technique, which they saw as useless against their defense plan, the gun.

Mike would simply ask these fantasy finger pointers, "What are you going to do? Shoot me with your finger?" Sometimes these nerds would actually respond, "No, I'd shoot you with a gun," making it necessary for Mike to point out the obvious: "But you don't have a gun."

Consider just how obvious it is that these people are in fantasy land with regard to the fact that they might really be attacked someday. In an important sense, their solution is to form a pistol with their hand and "shoot" the assailant. I won't dwell on this any further, but you might pause a bit and think on it some. With such a nonfunctional combat mind-set as this, even if these people did have a gun on them when attacked, it still might not do them any good. Can you see why?

Think about how denial works and when and why people engage in it. Also recognize why it is so naturally difficult to see it at work in ourselves.

ONE LEARNS TO FIGHT EMPTY-HANDED BECAUSE MOST TIMES, "THAT'S ALL YOU GOT"

Yeah, I know, I said this in *A Bouncer's Guide to Barroom Brawling*, but it bears repeating: the only reason for trying to defend yourself with your bare hands is simply because that's all you've got at the time—and the key phrase here may be *at the time*.

Police officers always carry handguns, yet many cops are stabbed to death with knives every year. Why? Well, if you were to ask a group of cops how they would respond to a knife attack, many might say, "I'd shoot the bastard."

This attitude reflects a failure in their training, because, had these officers experienced a scenario training program where a Bulletman-type assailant pulled a knife on them and attacked, they would immediately see that they could rarely get their guns out of their holsters before the Bulletman cut them up deep, wide, and handsome (as in, from belly to brisket).

Scenario training would show these officers that most times, in order to have a chance to draw their guns, they would first have to deal with the knife attack itself by stepping off the attack line and then using empty-handed defense. But in the absence of such training they don't realize this, and, thus believing that the gun is superior to the knife, they think, "I'll just shoot the bastard." Hence, a respectable number of armed police officers are killed with knives every year.

This is changing, however. I observe that more and more police forces are now engaging in some type of scenario-based training. Some officers tell me that it has already become the accepted method in some departments.

From my own instructional experience, I know that police in particular are often not very well motivated to learn empty-handed fighting techniques. But once they see that they can be stuck by the blade repeatedly before they can draw and fire their guns, then you have their attention.

A noted police firearms instructor once said to me quite flatly that there seemed to be no correlation at all between officers' shooting scores on the pistol range and their shooting performance on the street. When we consider that a police officer's firearms training may only have consisted of firing at paper targets, it should come as no surprise that we see no correlation. Why should we? The motor skills and hand-eye coordination one needs to hit targets on a range are only a fraction of what is required to blast lead through a man in an actual gunfight.

It is the same with classical martial arts training. Knowing how to throw a good, solid punch or execute any other technique in a dojo is not adequate for doing the same in a street fight. Consequently, cops don't shoot on the street like they shoot on the range, and martial artists don't fight on the street like they practice in the dojo. The primary reason for all this is fairly apparent. Their training does not adequately simulate the conditions found in the field. Most importantly, their training does not adequately simulate the visceral cues that elicit the adrenal stress reaction.

But in an actual combat incident, the introduction of adrenaline into the bloodstream is the one thing you can absolutely depend on. It is primarily how you handle that adrenaline reaction that will determine how effectively you will be able to use any weapon (including your bare hands).

Scenario Training Should Be Mandatory for Police

Personally, I think this type of training should be mandatory for police officers. It seems to be almost criminally negligent to put a gun in an officer's hand and then put him or her on the street without ever having performed under a real-life simulation of a potential lethal-force situation.

The scenario training method provides officers the opportunity to see how they would react. It would help weed out the bully types who panic and shoot at anything they perceive as a quick move on the part of the suspect. It would also provide the more mentally stable officer with the confidence level needed to enter into a potentially lethal situation and perform correctly and lawfully.

Fortunately, there now appears to be a greater recognition of this reality in police training, as the scenario method is being developed in some departments. Personally, I neither feel qualified nor am I especially interested in training police. Although we are all made of the same clay, police have some very special responsibilities that come with carrying a badge and gun that the ordinary citizen does not have.

Ironically, the cop, by necessity in a free society, must take greater risks in a confrontation than the ordinary citizen. This should be obvious. For example, preemption is a cardinal defensive strategy in my world, but a cop can't be drawing his gun every time things look a little hinky, much less whack somebody with a nightstick because he woofs on him hard.

Cops, particularly city cops, have a nearly impossible job on today's streets, and tomorrow's streets will certainly be even worse. The unfortunate but understandable result is a suicide, homicide, alcoholism, and divorce rate among cops that is many times the national average.

Therefore, any cop who does not take money or sell drugs, who does not habitually go badge-heavy and abuse his authority, and who will not protect a rapist, killer, or drug pusher because that person happens to carry a badge too, has my genuine respect. It is a job that I know I could not handle properly.

THERE IS JUST AS MUCH MISINFORMATION IN FIREARMS TRAINING AS THERE IS IN THE MARTIAL ARTS WORLD

In gun magazines, one can find the same type of undying controversies as are found in martial arts magazines. Instead of articles like, "Tae Kwon Do's Tornado Kicks vs. Shotokan's Circular Path to Victory," the gun magazines will run articles such as, "Point Shooting: Is There Any Point?" or "Weaver Stance vs. Instinct Shooting: Which is for You?"

In the martial arts world, most of the people writing the "how to fight" articles have never been in a real fight. Likewise, most of the authors of the gun books and magazine articles have never experienced a real shooting incident. If you doubt this, research the facts. You will find that of the top half-dozen "experts" putting out books or videos on defensive use of the handgun, only a few have ever actually shot anybody.

An Exception: Jeff Cooper's
Principles of Personal Defense

A notable exception to the rule would be Mr. Jeff Cooper, who has written (among other works) an excellent book titled *Principles of Personal Defense* (available from Paladin Press). In the 44 pages of this short work, Cooper conveys the essence of what I have tried to communicate both in this book and in my last. Does he dwell on shooting stances, choice of handguns, loads, sights, or gun leather? No, he does not. The book deals with the nature and psychology of the "predator" assailant and the mind-set you need to defeat him. Cooper makes the following very significant point about the criminal assailant: "As we have seen, what he usually least suspects is instant, violent counterattack." (Get this book and read it.)

My point is that it's primarily those people who have no combat experience that will argue endlessly and vehemently about what are actually very trivial matters concerning stance, sights, weapon type, and so on. This is basically the same thing as martial artists who have never been in a fight debating over why one style is superior to another.

However, once someone has actually experienced the adrenal effects of combat, all these matters are generally put in their proper perspective. This is because the real challenge of actual combat is just that—dealing effectively with those adrenal effects. Once this is understood (which means experienced), discussions about style, technique, and so on can sound like arguments over how many angels can dance on the head of a pin.

Hence, a real-life gunfighter such as Jeff Cooper doesn't waste much ink on talking about which gun to use in what caliber or which stance is best in *Principles of Personal Defense*. Instead, he addresses the real problem—understanding your enemy and what he expects, and thus why your attitude can be more decisive than your weapon in determining who is left alive.

THE PROBLEM WITH EXPERIENCE AND DOGMATISM

The first time someone tried to kill me with a knife was a somewhat mind-altering experience. My assailant likely expected that I would choke when first cut, but I had another response programmed into me, and I immediately controlled the weapon hand and then pounded the hell out of the guy with my free hand. I drove him across the floor to keep his balance broken (knocking over tables, chairs, and bar patrons) until I slammed him into the wall, whereupon I continued to break his clavicles, his nose, and so on. If there really is such a thing as luck, I must have had plenty of it not to have had my medical record closed in that incident.

Here's the point: if, shortly after this attack, someone in a martial arts dojo, dojang, or kwoon had tried to show me some esoteric knife defense, I doubt that I would have been at all receptive to absorbing that instruction. My mind would have had difficulty getting past the traumatic reality of my having been cut and having seen my blood all over everywhere. Add to all this the blinding speed with which everything had happened, and you can see why I would have been very unlikely to have any confidence at all in the movements the instructor was demonstrating. They would have seemed simply irrelevant or even suicidal to me when measured against the personal experience of a real-world knife attack.

Therefore, it would have been easy for me to say, "Give it up, man. You'll never have time to even think about all that stuff—you just gotta grab that knife hand and drive the bastard across the floor until he slams into some shit, then beat the hell out of him."

Beginning to get the idea? Such incidents tend to make one's thinking rather dogmatic concerning the correct way to handle them. I think this is one of the "artifacts" of adrenal stress. Occasionally, I have had the chance (one I seek out when appropriate and possible) to discuss combat incidents with people who have experienced them. The incident may have been a bar fight, a policeman's experience in a shooting incident, or a military combat situation. For the most part, a fight is a fight.

Sometimes these people are firearms instructors or "hand-to-hand" fighting instructors who will insist that a particular way of handling a given attack is THE ONLY WAY. That's in all capital letters, you see, as in, "if you try any other way in dealing with the situation, you are a fool who has just purchased an express ticket to the morgue."

One can see the impatience in their faces and the frustration in their voices that come from a perception of being unable to communicate to someone what to them is an obvious truth—because that person has not had a combat experience similar to theirs. Their experience, in which they used the aforementioned technique or approach that saved their lives, causes them to become zealot advocates of the given approach or technique because of the adrenal effects of combat.

Ironically, the adrenal effect has very likely left them with a distorted memory of what actually happened anyway. I think there are cases where they may not have even used the technique or approach that they trained on and "know" they used in the combat incident. To the contrary, they may have done something entirely spontaneous—not what they trained on at all—that actually saved them. But they may recall having performed as they were trained because that is their only rational context within which to frame the adrenal event.

Your humble narrator has likely been guilty on occasion of this kind of thinking, too. We try to piece together the fragments of our memory of an event involving adrenal stress. But, almost like in a dream, those fragments often don't make any sense to our conscious and rational minds. Therefore, our minds try to enforce some sense or rationality on them after the fact. This can lead an individual to the certain belief as to what happened, which is actually a "false memory."

An example we see in the weapons course from time to time occurs when a person has been trained in, say, a Weaver or isosceles stance for combat use of the pistol. Sometimes these people will succeed in drawing the weapon in time and will fire the two rounds into the assailant's head or center of body mass in their first scenario. But when we ask them to recall what they did in the scenario, they will say something like, "I saw him draw the weapon and I drew my pistol, assumed a Weaver stance, and immediately fired two shoots into him as he closed."

Sounds pretty good, huh? In fact, they actually did draw and fire effectively because they put the rounds on target before they were "killed." But, when they see the videotape of themselves, they see that they did not use any kind of "Weaver" stance, or "isosceles" stance, or anything else. They just jerked out the pistol and shot the guy. Again, it is the adrenal stress that confuses their memory of events.

Keep this in mind when studying with a dogmatic instructor who teaches the method that "saved his life in the deadly encounter." The method he "knows" he used and now instructs may be only a confused recollection created by the adrenal stress of the event.

Many of the traditional training methods in the defensive use of the pistol have no more relevance to actual combat use of the pistol than martial arts training methods have to a real street fight. These standard pistol training methods have some value, but they do not engage the real problem, and this is why they leave the shooter so poorly prepared for an actual encounter.

There is always more than one way to deal with a given combat situation, and dogmatic thinking is closed-minded thinking, which always has at its root some kind of *fear*.

Before leaving this idea of how a combat experience can lead to an inflexible attitude or even an irrational instructional approach, let me say that I am always interested in hearing how somebody else survived a real combat experience and lived to tell the tale, and so should you be. To repeat the opening line of *A Bouncer's Guide,* "Training is useful, but it is no substitute for experience."

An Experiment in Adapting Scenario-Based Training to the Combat Use of the Pistol

This experiment was conducted early in the development of our pistol course. We selected six people who had taken our basic course (hand-to-hand fighting) but had never handled a real firearm in their lives. Later, we selected a second group of six people who were "regular" shooters and owned pistols. They had not taken our basic course.

The basic course people were given 90 seconds of instruction in the use of the Smith & Wesson 586 revolver. This consisted of a demonstration of how to open and close the cylinder, and they all dry-fired the weapon. They passed the weapon from one person to the next, each one pointing the gun at the ceiling and pulling the trigger twice to get used to the trigger pull.

The experienced shooters viewed a 17-minute videotape that explained the scenario training methodology and showed some Bulletman fight scenarios a few days before they participated in the experiment.

Both groups were given the same scenario instructions. They were told that in this scenario they were on their own property or at their place of work (premises under their control) but were not actually in their house or inside their office or workplace.

Examples were given, such as they had just parked their car on the street and were walking to their front door, or they were taking some trash to the Dumpster in the alley directly outside their place of work.

They were told that their possession of the pistol was lawful but that they would have to justify any use of it under the law. The "law" was that they were not to draw or display the weapon until they determined that an attack was clearly imminent or actually in progress. At that point, they were to fire two shots into the center of mass of the assailant. I pounded my fist over my sternum to demonstrate where their shots were to be placed.

Both groups got about the same level of attack speed, which was full speed. The Bulletman was simply told to try to get them. Only edged weapons were used in the attacks. These were the knife, machete, and meat cleaver. (The rubber weapons we use look pretty real.)

The pistol was loaded with two "cartridges," which were indexed to come up on the first two pulls of the trigger. These were actually primed .38-caliber shells loaded with rubber bullets. There was no gunpowder; only the primer propelled the rubber bullets, firing them with enough velocity to break the skin of exposed flesh and holding a reasonably accurate line of aim out to 30 feet or more.

The pistol-retention system was the same for everyone. We provided a large leather belt with extra holes punched into it so it could be adjusted to the user's individual waist size. The pistol was then slipped under the belt in the small of the back or slightly to the side. This is sometimes referred to in gun literature as the "Mexican" carry (for reasons unknown to me).

The results of these scenarios were that the basic course graduates did much better that the "experienced" shooters. They scored more lethal hits and were "killed" far less often than those with previous handgun experience. In particular, of the six basic course graduates, all managed to draw the weapon and retreat off the attack line while firing two shots at the closing Bulletman. There was one misfire; otherwise, only two of the 12 bullets fired missed the Bulletman. Five of the six basic course graduates put bullets into the chest area of the assailant. The sixth graduate fired twice, striking the Bulletman once in the arm. However, it did happen to be the assailant's weapon arm (he was wielding a machete), so the fighter was judged to have survived the encounter. The machete never touched him.

The experienced shooters' performance was a different story entirely. Only one of these shooters placed both rounds in the chest of the assailant before the assailant made contact with him. Two failed to get the gun out or fire before they were overtaken by the closing Bulletman and "killed" with a knife. One failed to get off any shots because he fumbled the weapon on the draw and dropped it to the mat. The fifth shooter invalidated his scenario by drawing the weapon prematurely, that is, before there was any demonstrated justifiable cause. When given a second scenario he drew and scored one hit to the chest. The sixth member of this group did not show up the night we conducted this experiment.

Several weeks later, two of the experienced shooters were given a similar version of the scenario experiment, and both did much better. I have little doubt that in a day they would have been doing as well as or better than the basic course graduates. But the point is, before this experiment was conducted, had these people been attacked for real in circumstances similar to the scenario we gave them, I believe they would have performed much like they did in that first scenario.

Yet the experience of the experiment itself, which exposed them to some amount of adrenal stress as well as allowing them to watch the other scenarios go down, apparently had quite a significant amount of instructional value for them. This is why the two guys did so much better weeks later.

The problems the experienced shooters had in the scenarios were the direct result of adrenal effects. The dropping of the gun by one of these individuals appeared to me to be a clear result of a partial loss of fine motor control coupled with his overamped effort to get the gun out immediately. The results of our experiment echo of the aforementioned police firearms instructor's observation that there seemed to be no correlation between officers' shooting performance on the pistol range and their shooting performance on the street.

Clearly, the difference between our experienced shooters' performance when shooting at targets on the pistol range and that when shooting at the Bulletman in the scenario can only be attributed the differences in the adrenalization level under which the two activities were carried out.

On the other hand, I believe that a fighter's performance in a scenario under the effects of adrenalization reflects with much more accuracy how he or she might perform in an actual combat situation, be it with a gun, a knife, a stick, or empty-handed.

Further, each additional fight scenario the fighter experiences enhances the likelihood that he or she will deal with an actual attack the same way. It also seems

DYNAMIC "POINT SHOOTING" SCENARIOS

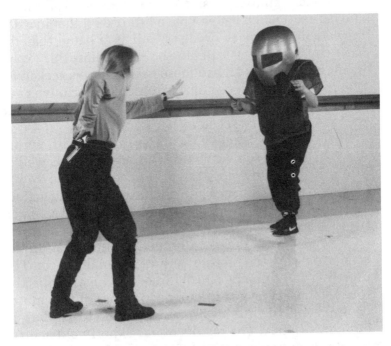

This exercise begins with the fighter's eyes closed. Starting out with the eyes closed increases the adrenal anxiety and better simulates the surprise of an actual situation. She is armed with a Model 586 Smith & Wesson .357 Magnum revolver, which is loaded with rubber bullets. When she opens her eyes she must evaluate and deal with whatever situation she finds herself facing. In this case she immediately sees a man with a knife in his hands. Knowing that a man with a knife can very quickly close the distance and kill, she draws the pistol immediately and commands him to "halt!"

apparent that it is the first three or four fight scenarios that make the most dramatic difference in performance.

Some Observations about Our
Scenario-Based Pistol Training

Just as the fight scenarios allow martial arts people to discover the problems in applying their technique, likewise, firearms people discover problems in their shooting technique when they must perform under adrenal stress and hit a living, moving assailant.

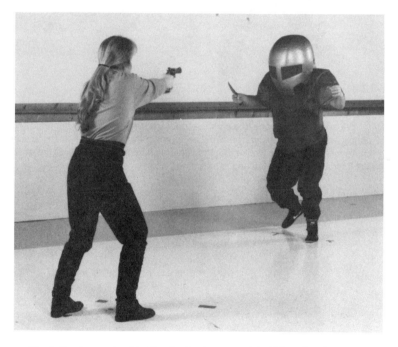

The knifer does not halt but begins to charge, and the fighter fires immediately. The first rubber bullet strikes the assailant in the head, and this would very likely stop the attacker. However, since handgun bullets are not the "instant" stoppers that movies and TV would lead us to believe, the assailant continues his charge without pause. But the fighter has not stopped shooting and at this point has fired two more rubber bullets into him.

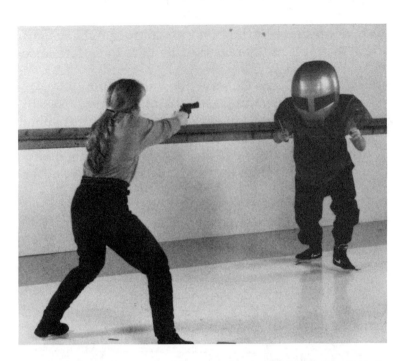

We are now about one and a half seconds into the assailant's attempted knife attack, and he has been hit by the rubber bullets three times. Still, he continues his charge with the blade. Notice that the fighter is beginning to move off the attack line (in this case, to her left and to the corner).

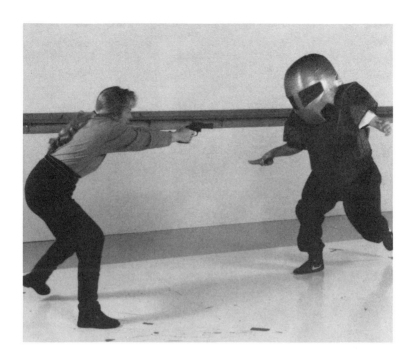

The fighter's moving to the corner and off the attack line forces the charging knifer to have to turn in midcharge. This buys the defender another critical half second for target acquisition, and she fires a fourth round into her assailant.

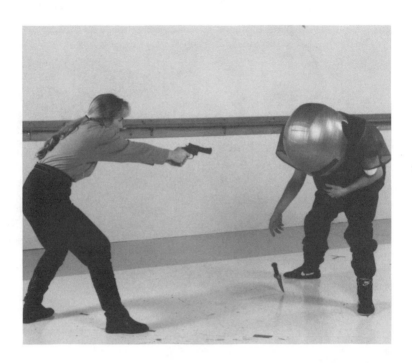

Her fifth round again hits the assailant in the center of mass, and his charge falters. The defender then fires her sixth and final round into his head, and the assailant drops the knife and collapses. This is an example of a dynamic "point shooting" scenario. The sights of the weapon are never engaged, both eyes are kept open and on the enemy, and she puts all six bullets into the attacker. Statistics show that most shootings in the real world occur at distances of 8 feet or less. Point shooting techniques, with some practice, are effective and accurate to distances of at least 25 feet.

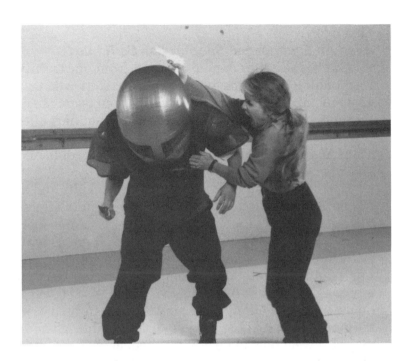

In this exercise the gun fails to fire (a malfunction—a round is not chambered or the safety is still on) or the bullets simply fail to stop the attack. The fighter must instantly make the transition to hand-to-hand techniques. She moves immediately to the nonweapon side of the assailant , slaps down his attempt at a grab, strikes him behind the neck with the pistol with full force, and runs past him, opening the distance as she clears the pistol and gets it into action.

Lesson #1:
Even An Experienced Shooter Can Be Rattled

One lesson that can be gleaned from our training methodology concerns experienced shooters who try to give the impression that the scenarios aren't going to rattle them before they actually undergo that part of the training. First, allow me to relate the conditions of the scenarios where these "I won't be rattled" people often give themselves away.

If, for instance, the Bulletman draws a knife and the fighter chooses not to kill him at once, then the fighter has been instructed to say, "Drop the knife now or I'll shoot!" With some frequency, I notice that the "it won't rattle me" people have drawn their pistol and are pointing it at the Bulletman before the Bulletman has done anything to warrant it. (In the real world, their behavior might support a felony menacing charge.) In such cases, the gun is often shaking, as is the fighter. If the fighter displays his weapon and he doesn't shoot at once, he forgets all about verbally commanding the behavior he wants, such as, "Drop the knife." Instead, he shouts things like, "Stay there—don't come any closer."

It isn't my intent to make fun of these people. After all, if everybody did it right the first time, there would be no need for this training. But this type of behavior shows that these people are at least partially overcome by adrenal stress and fear and are not really in control of themselves. This also makes them much more likely to shoot prematurely or shoot someone by accident in a real-life situation.

The scenario gives them some experience with the situation of holding a gun on someone under adrenal stress and making that critical "shoot/don't shoot" decision.

Lesson #2:
They Have to See It to Believe It

Another valuable lesson that these scenarios show shooters who are used to hitting the paper targets at the range with speed and accuracy (maybe even out to 25 yards or so) is that under adrenal stress they can miss at three or four feet. Until they experience this, it's all but pointless to try to convince them that it can even happen. (Indeed, we do a lot less verbal instruction now than we did in our first few years of using this adrenal stress scenario-based training methodology. Now, we primarily let them experience the problem, and we just try to use verbal expression to help them put it into context.) Without the adrenal stress factor, experienced shooters would never miss a paper target at such a close range, even if they fired as fast as they could. Still, they often miss the Bulletman.

Clearly, the difference in performance between shooting at targets on the pistol range and shooting at the Bulletman in the scenario can only be attributed to the differences in the adrenalization level under which the two activities were carried out.

THE PRIMARY GOAL OF SCENARIO TRAINING WITH WEAPONS: DEVELOPING THE PROPER MIND-SET

Some people in our weapons program need assistance in getting past what may be a natural reluctance on the part of a decent person to use a knife or other weapon on another human being. To address this, a training method we use when teaching the basics of using a knife for self-defense (referred to as the fundamentals of "slicing, sticking, and gutting") is as follows.

Taking out two or three real knives, I will expose the blades of the weapons, and then they are passed around to each of the fighters, who are sitting in a circle. A speech such as the following is given:

> Okay, I want you to examine the blades, hold them in your hands, get the feel of them, experiment with both grips [demonstrations of "ice pick" and "sabre" grips are given], and I want you to imagine the circumstances that would compel you to use this weapon on another human being

with the intent to stop and/or kill him. For some of you it might be something like, "Well, if somebody broke into my house and was attacking my kid, then I'd kill him with the knife before I saw him kill my kid."

I want you to visualize your using the knife under these circumstances to kill such a person. After you have had a few minutes to think about it, we are all going to discuss what those circumstances might be.

There are some other parts to this, but it ultimately comes down to everyone explaining a circumstance wherein they would be prepared to use the knife to kill somebody. Most times there are a few people—often but not exclusively women—who say something like, "I know I have a right to defend myself, but I'm just not sure I could really do it, actually cut somebody like that."

My response is, "I understand. It is a reflection of your decency and humanity that brings you to think like that, but don't worry. As the course progresses you will see that you would be more than capable of using the knife in this manner if it was really demanded of you. However, you do need to have a few ideas about how to use the blade effectively and how to retain the blade from the attempted disarm, so that's what we are going to look at first."

Later, when the course has progressed to the point of the fight scenarios (which are made even more intense for weapons training), adrenalization turns these people who said that they were "just not sure they could ever cut anybody" into full-on Freddy Kruegers on holiday. We do a videotape analysis of the fights, and it's a real hoot to play the voice of the person saying, "I just don't know if I could actually use a knife on another person; I just don't think I could do it" while watching her image on the TV screen straddling a fallen Bulletman, holding the knife with both hands, and screaming as she makes repeated and powerful downward thrust into his chest and face.

Kind of gets me all misty-eyed just thinking about it. So before I go all mushy on you, I'll just get on with it.

Adrenal stress tends to actualize brain functions that occur on a baser level than normal, conscious thought. It's not the "me" inside you that is thinking about the ethical issues or is squeamish about cutting somebody who is using the knife in the scenarios. It is the "animal" inside of the "me." It's like that animal inside is saying, "I'm taking over now before you get us both killed."

The woman who discovers she can use the weapon, that she does have the instinct and will to survive, has set up an emergency communication line with that beast within. Under the adrenal stress of an actual attack, she will dial up "beast girl," who will take over immediately.

Sometimes you can see that mental transformation take place in people. It shows that clearly in their faces. An example is when you see a woman (we'll call her Jane) who holds the knife in her hand between classes and looks at in a way that clearly reflects a dawning confidence born of her realization and conviction that she really could defeat an assailant. It as if you hear her thoughts say, "Damn, with this I really would have a chance." I visualize this woman humming along pleasantly in her kitchen slicing potatoes for the evening meal when Mr. Serial Rapist busts through her back door looking for rape/murder victim number four.

Then, he meets our little Jane and dies in shocked disbelief, spitting blood as she stabs him about seven times in the gut before he can even try to grab the knife. When he does try to grab Jane's knife hand she gives him the quick "knife twirl" that severs all the major structures on the inside of his wrist and immediately returns with the old thrust to the carotid artery after having knocked his head back with a sweet palm heel strike that sets up the perfect angle.

Well, there I go, waxing sentimental again.

But as far as little Jane is concerned, all that people have to do to avoid being gutted like this in her kitchen is to not try to break in and rape and murder her. They better leave her family alone, too. This seems perfectly reasonable to me, and, frankly, I enjoy training people to deal with these type criminals in this fashion.

The knife is a very deadly weapon, equal to the firearm in some circumstances. Equally important, once you get their minds right (the combat mind-set), everyone can learn very quickly to use the knife in a way that is extremely difficult for the assailant who is expecting a victim to defend against successfully.

The knife is also the weapon a person is most likely to have access to—more so than the gun in most cases. Right now, as you are reading this book, how quickly could you get a knife in your hand? Now, how quickly could you get a gun in your hand? For some, one just means a trip to the kitchen but the other might mean unlocking a gun safe or maybe even a visit to the gun shop itself (maybe even a five-day waiting period or more after that).

If a person is reluctant to train realistically in the use of deadly weapons such as the knife or gun, it suggests to me that they have not truly accepted the reality that they may have to use lethal force someday to survive. Such an attitude naturally tends to make me doubt their combat mind-set and thus their unarmed fighting ability in a real attack as well.

The fact is that any altercation between two or more human beings always has the potential for a homicide, weapons or not. Fighting is not normal, civilized behavior. Once things get physically primitive, even what might be called "natural homicidal forces" can be set loose. Once violence begins it's often, as Shakespeare put it, "Cry, 'Havoc'! and let slip the dogs of war."

Again, I recall what Stephen Hayes said to me about the objective of self-defense. He said its objective was to make someone stop doing something. For example, stop trying to beat me up, or rape me, or attack my family, etc. Ultimately, Mr. Hayes said that the thing the attacker might have to stop doing is living.

I think this expresses it very well.

If you have difficulty visualizing yourself using a

knife on a person or shooting them to defend your life, then you need to work on your understanding of these things. A decent person does not want to hurt or kill anyone. But sometimes this is what you may have to do to save your life or that of a loved one. You had best prepare for that both physically and mentally now—it may be too late when an attack actually occurs.

Failure to do such mental preparation and to absorb some basic techniques for self-defense will significantly reduce your chances of survival in a crisis. Ignoring or denying the fact that these things could happen to you won't help either. It will only leave you more vulnerable. It's as simple as that.

EXTRAORDINARY MARTIAL SKILL WITH THE WEAPON IS NOT DEMANDED TO SURVIVE MOST REAL-WORLD ATTACKS

Some time ago I had a brief encounter with a very good knife fighting instructor and quite a polished martial artist in general, Mr. James Keating. When I saw this guy do his knife-in-each-hand, "siniwali"-type drill, his knives seemed to move a lot like the blades on a food blender, only a little faster. It is very difficult for me to imagine someone surviving a stand-up knife fight with this guy.

There is no "posing" with this dude, either. He knows how to use those blades, but he is a level-headed, decent guy who would never bully anyone or use violence unless it was truly forced on him. He is also, I believe, a seventh-degree black belt in goju-ryu karate. After getting a little visual taste of his skill with the steel, I asked him why he chose to specialize in the knife. His response was simply that the knife is the weapon a person is most likely to have on him when attacked.

I must agree, the knife is the weapon you most likely will be able to carry. Thus, it is the weapon most likely to benefit you in a real-world life-and-death fight. Not only is Mr. Keating very good with the blade, but since that encounter I have observed that he knows something about how to instruct as well.

When I asked him if he felt it was really necessary to develop the level of skill that he had achieved in order to be able to defend oneself using a knife, he acknowledged at once that it was not. In fact, he said, "Anybody with a knife is dangerous."

As I recall, he also basically agreed that the Hollywood scenario of two guys squaring off and circling each other in a knife fight (that is, both having knives) is not the most likely one for a knife incident. But he also acknowledged that this can happen, and, in fact, he had experienced such an incident himself.

The point here is that most of the knife arts (the most combat-effective, to my knowledge, being the Filipino and silat styles) concentrate on developing techniques for fighting another guy who has a knife and knows how to use it. But that's not the most likely scenario for most people, especially here in the United States.

Most of the martial technique studied in knife fighting courses are more technique than is required for a person to be able to use a blade in the most likely self-defense situations he might face—particularly when he takes the initiative with the weapon on the typical street mugger who has already selected him as a "victim."

To return to the immediate point, Mr. Keating's level of skill with the blade, while enviable, is not required to be able to use a knife effectively for your own self-defense (in all but some very rare situations). Again, it is my belief that to use any weapon effectively in combat, you first need to have proper combat mind-set and thus act decisively and without hesitation. This all comes back to what every true master I have ever dealt with has acknowledged—namely that you don't need a lot of techniques for real-world self-defense.

Mr. Keating told me that while he recognized that it was unlikely that he would ever have to face someone with his level of training or skill in a knife fight, this was precisely the person he was training to deal with.

There can be no challenge to this logic, particularly for someone with Mr. Keating's level of talent. But few people are born with such talent or will ever develop such skill. (Be that as it may, if you are serious about learning the finer points of using a knife in combat, I recommend you go see Mr. Keating.)

SCENARIO TRAINING USING THE STICK

The stick or club has got to be mankind's first weapon. The Filipino arts of arnis and kali are the predominate martial arts that focus on the stick. Persons more knowledgeable of these arts might say that much of this Filipino stick work is really meant for the short bolo machete. This is true, but the many of the mechanics of using a machete are closer to those of a stick than a short knife.

In any case, a stick is not a weapon equal to the gun or the knife. Also, the Filipino arts assume the other guy has a stick or knife as well, and a lot of the technique is predicated on this assumption of weapon versus weapon. It is a lot easier when you are the only one with a stick, particularly if the closing enemy is taken by surprise with the weapon.

In our scenario-based training we do not get into complex stick work; we concentrate on power and accuracy in a nontelegraphed strike and continuous attack.

Imagine this scenario: you have a good stick in your hand, and the aggressor is woofing on you and closing the distance.

Are you confident that you can step off the attack line and strike a single powerful blow that will disable him long enough (like one second) for you to strike a second, more damaging blow, followed by a third and fourth, and so on? Keep in mind that if your first strike does not take him out or hurt him enough for the follow-up shots, then you will find yourself in a standing grapple, and at this point your stick will be much less useful as a weapon. In fact, you might be disarmed of the stick, and then he can use it on you.

To strike that opening blow with power and accuracy and in a way that occurs so explosively that the enemy cannot "read" the strike and thus reduce the impact by an evasion is not a skill we are born with. We are only born with the survival instinct; *how* we survive has to be learned.

To strike such a blow certainly does not take years of study, but on the other hand, how many untrained people do you think can do this *the first time out* in a Bulletman scenario? The correct answer is less than half. How many in an actual confrontation? I submit that even fewer persons would succeed the first time out against a determined assailant in a real attack.

On the other hand, after a few simple drills and a scenario or two, most everyone can do it. Actually, there really is not a great deal that has to be taught (a few particulars about getting real power, use of hip rotation, and so on) before sending people into the fight scenarios. This is because all it takes is a little footwork and a proper reading of the assailant's attack or charge. For the most part, people learn to do it themselves simply by experiencing the scenarios. They can feel and hear when their shot is correct, and they can also feel it when they strike only a glancing blow. It's not that difficult; it's just that generally people just don't get this kind of practice hitting a person in the head with a stick full force when that person is woofing on them and then makes his surprise attack.

After a short time the fighters are striking only the bone-cracking beauty shots that would drop most people straight off. Consider that this is only after about an hour or less of training. I do not know of any other training method that could achieve this result consistently. The scenario method of training allows the fighters to learn to do it by doing it, and they get immediate feedback on the quality and effectiveness of each strike they make in a dynamic, moving scenario.

I have seen women who never thought about "fighting" at all learn to use the stick so well that they actually use feints and baits that they make up themselves on the spot to set up the assailant for a full-blown beauty shot to the face. This is not common, but I have seen it occur. Hell, their fake-outs even fool me sometimes when I'm watching the fights.

Now if one of these women had a tire iron or other stick-type weapon in her hand and an actual assailant was confronting her, it is highly possible that the assailant might not see her "stick" as any real threat and hence just come right on in, assuming he would easily disarm her. What a surprise would be in store for him as he saw those purple lights against that black background before that final "fade to black."

My contention is that simply having rehearsed the action of striking a person in the head with the stick with full power as he charges in on you in an adrenal stress-driven scenario dramatically increases the probability that you will strike an effective blow in a real-world attack.

Keep in mind that a stick is a less "offensive" weapon than a gun or knife to police or the courts. This means you might be able to have one handy in a situation where a gun or knife might not be acceptable for legal reasons. Look around you—what could be used as a stick in a crisis?

The Dog Brothers

In closing this section on scenario-based training with the stick, I must include a mention of the "Dog Brothers," aka Marc Denny and Eric Knaus in Hermosa Beach, California.

To give it to you short and sweet, these guys came howling out of the Dan Inosanto Academy in Los Angeles with a good grasp of jeet kune do and the Filipino stick and knife arts of kali and arnis.

At some point they looked at each other and said something like, "Yeah, but what would happen if we really hit each other with the sticks, using the minimum of protective gear such that the blows would hurt enough to get a realistic response from the hit?"

If you look closely at Denny's "Crafty Dog" business

card, you'll see small graphics depicted in each corner of a triangle. These graphics represent mind, heart, and balls. On a spiritual level, it requires all three to step up to the annual "gathering of the pack" in Hermosa Beach for the "fights" in the park. What I want you to appreciate is that these guys are not machismo assholes; they don't really do this to show how tough they are. They do it to explore the warrior spirit and to exercise same in a way that few martial arts people are willing to step up for.

They hit full contact with the sticks (Denny prefers the term "real contact"), using only light fencing masks and some sort of gloves, generally lighter than hockey gloves.

Blood is spilled, but these men keep to the only rule of the game, which is, "Everyone leaves friends at the end of the day." There are no cheap shots or attempts to hit the opponent with a damaging blow when he is unable to defend himself from a previous "head ringer" or if he has lost his protection (gets the fencing mask knocked off his head).

This level of contact is certainly not for everybody, but it is something that everybody can watch and learn from if he or she has an open mind. The Dog Brothers have some videotapes out, and they now teach some stick fighting seminars around the country. (Their videotape *Real Contact Stick Fighting* is available through Paladin Press.)

I have no doubt that either of these guys would be a terror in a real fight, even if he did not have a stick in his hand, because their training method tests, develops, and strengthens the warrior spirit of "entering in" and "striking down the enemy."

A FINAL NOTE: THE MOST DANGEROUS ASSAILANTS DON'T DISPLAY THEIR WEAPONS BEFORE USING THEM

My own attitude toward this subject is colored by my having been present when two people, neither of which had any time to draw a blade in their own defense, were murdered with knives in two separate incidents. Yet I believe they both could have survived if they had been more aware and in control of themselves. Improper combat attitude killed them as surely as did the blade.

Of course, having been attacked with knives and having been cut up a bit myself has left an impression on me as well—both mental and physical.

Most of the times I saw somebody draw a knife in my bar work, it was defensively, that is, to keep people from coming after them (attacking). Perhaps there is no truly typical example of this, but the image that comes to mind is when one guy punches out the other and knocks him to the floor. Then the punch-out victim jumps up, opens his knife, and, displaying it openly, yells out something like, "Don't fuck with me, motherfucker, or I'll cut you, man!"

The guy displaying the knife like this seldom intends to attack with the blade. He is using the blade to discourage the guy who punched him out from continuing the festivities and to show that he is prepared to use lethal force rather than be beat up further. He is also using the weapon to save face, because although the guy punched him out, he is hoping to demonstrate (to himself and the multitude) that now, this guy is not willing to face him when he's got a blade in his hand. He is thus not "impotent."

This dangerous child displaying the weapon for show is in contrast to the true homicidal knifer, who will almost never allow the victim to see the blade before he uses it to lethal effect.

During one of the knife killings I witnessed, nobody ever even saw a knife or knew anyone had been stabbed until the victim started staggering and then fell down dead. The other case was almost too bizarre to relate. The victim had deliberately parachuted into a large biker party in an open field when some scooter trash cut out a piece of his parachute as a "mojo" or souvenir. The parachutist had to go "macho man" and run up to punch the guy out. Not very good tactical thinking, running up to punch out a guy who has a knife in his hands. It cost the parachutist his life. Still, nobody could report having seen the actual stabbing. There was quite a crowd to obscure the view, and things happened almost instantly.

On balance, while every situation must be dealt with on its individual merits, if things were to come to the point that I had to use a knife on somebody, it is unlikely that I would display the knife before I cut him. Nor would I be particularly likely to use the knife as a threat. If I had to use a knife or any other deadly weapon, it would only be because my life (or that of my wife, good pals, or anyone who owes me money) was in imminent danger. In such a case, one's first use of the weapon must be decisive.

It is a mistaken mind-set to think too much about the deterrent value of a given weapon. First off, if you display your knife or pistol as a threat, the other guy may draw a gun and shoot you dead. Even if this does not happen, in displaying your weapon you have lost the element of surprise, and if he does attack he will do so knowing you have the weapon.

Some people will attack even though their intended victim draws a pistol on them and orders them to "stay where they are" or be shot. Sometimes when the assailant attacks under these circumstances he is shot . . . and sometimes the victim chokes and is disarmed and then shot with his own weapon.

Consider why somebody would continue to attack a person who was holding a gun on them and had declared his intention to shoot if attacked? Why would someone still attack in the face of the deadly weapon? The only answer is because he doesn't think the person will shoot him. If this sounds hard to believe, consider that the assailant has already chosen the person he is attacking as a victim, and in his mind he has already succeeded as predator. Thus it may be that he can't immediately accept the new view of what's happening. He denies the situation because "victims don't do this." He continues to attack almost because he can't help himself. (For some documentation on this phenomenon, read *Handgun Stopping Power,* available from Paladin Press).

People who think that the menacing or dangerous looks of a gun or knife will have a deterrent such that they won't have to use the weapon are living in a state of denial similar to the aforementioned assailant. Further, such a mind-set makes it a) much more likely that they will never get their weapon in their hands before they are killed, and b) much more likely that they will be disarmed and killed should they live to display their weapon as a "deterrent." This is because they have improper combat mind-set.

In our bar work and at other times, both Mike Haynack, the Mad Chinaman, and I have disarmed people of knives and, in a few cases, pistols. In one case, the pistol came off a plainclothes cop who was beating up a woman on the boardwalk of New Jersey when Mike, the Amazing Eagle, felt compelled to intercede.

Back in those days (and hopefully now if it ever came up again), when I saw the weapon I'd disarm the person immediately, or I'd already be dead. More importantly, if I didn't go for it right then I figured I still might be dead. This is not to say I wouldn't jump over the bar or such to defend against a weapon attack by evading it. This is choice number one when possible. But if I couldn't escape like that, I'd blast and disarm immediately and on reflex.

To put this into real-world terms for you, while there are some circumstances where one might use the display of a weapon to effectively discourage an attack (and I admit to having done so a few times), to display your weapon is to give away your strongest tactical advantage which is the effective surprise use of the weapon.

Think about this realistically and do not assume that just because you draw a knife or gun that the other guys will give it up. They may draw their own gun or knife and kill you immediately, or they may disarm you immediately and kill you with your own weapon. It is most often a mistake to draw a deadly weapon unless you are prepared to kill with it without hesitation as required. There are people who will immediately see any hesitation in your eyes and will then close immediately for the disarm.

Also, make yourself knowledgeable about the law in your area about the use of lethal force and the carry of weapons. In general, outside your own home, if you use a gun on somebody it's going to very likely cause big legal problems. Almost unbelievably, in some states it can cause you big legal problems even if you are in your own home when somebody forces entry and you shoot him.

Beyond all this, if you have proper combat mind-set, which means control of adrenal stress, you are far less likely to shoot someone you did not intend to shoot in a crisis situation. I believe this is perhaps the principal benefit of scenario-based, adrenal conditioning training using the firearm.

My advice is to think about all this before you face such a situation. In fact, think about this before you decide to obtain a gun or carry a blade. Imagine the situations that could occur which might force you to use the weapon and how you would handle it. These mental rehearsals are not just a game. They can be very valuable—even life-saving—tools, so experiment with them realistically. If you discover that you cannot visualize yourself cutting someone's throat to save your life or a family member's life, then you have discovered a "problem" area you need to work on. Do this work before your life or a family member's life rides on your field performance.

Some Final
Thoughts

Throughout this text, I have demonstrated how the scenario-based training methodology allows us to channel the positive effects of adrenal stress in order to increase a person's chances of survival in an actual life-and-death encounter. I have also touched on the negative effects of adrenal stress and how they can interfere with a person's functioning effectively under such circumstances. Many people have asked me, "Can any training program work to *control the dysfunctional effects* of adrenal stress in a combat situation?" Based on my experience with the scenario-based training methodology, my answer to this is a simple "yes," while acknowledging that no training program can guarantee the field performance of the fighter. All we can do is increase people's odds by actualizing their full potential for survival. This is primarily accomplished by conditioning them to the adrenal reaction so that they are far less likely to choke and thus can respond and make use of any technical training they may have in that first critical second of a life-threatening encounter.

Still, there are some people with combat experience who instruct what I see as basically good programs which take the position that the adrenal effect will be certain and severe and therefore the training method must recognize and accept this. This attitude might express itself in a pistol training program that advocates the isosceles stance, which has the arms locked and fully extended, over the Weaver-type stance, which requires finer motor control. The logic here would be that the "natural thing" for a person to do in a gunfight is to freeze up a bit and thrust his arms straight out in front of him while pointing the gun at the enemy in a tight grip. Therefore (as this way of thinking goes), since this is what people are going to do anyway, it's best that we train them to shoot effectively in that position.

I believe that there is some clear logic to this thinking. But, it is not my purpose to suggest that the isosceles stance is more functional than the Weaver stance. This depends on the individual shooter and the particular circumstances of the gunfight. How important is stance anyway in a real gunfight?

The point I am trying to make is that the logic of constructing a training methodology that builds on what people are already known to do naturally under stress is a sound one. For example, the inside and outside crane technique for slipping a blow and immediately returning a counterstrike (which was a major subject of *Bouncer's Guide*) partly originates from this logic. The natural thing to do when someone takes a swing at your head is to throw your hands up in front of your face and turn your head away. The crane technique simply polishes this natural reaction into a reflex that more effectively slips the blow and sets up the counterstrike.

But I strongly disagree with the idea that sometimes accompanies this "train them the way they naturally respond to stress" position—namely, that you can't train people successfully to deal with adrenal stress itself. The assumption here is that some people will panic no matter what and only a few won't, because that's just their individual nature, and training can't really change that. I know that this is not the case.

How individuals respond to the adrenal stress of a real-world attack will depend very significantly on their antecedent experience with this biochemistry. People can develop a tolerance to adrenaline in the same way they do to alcohol, heroin, or any other drug. This tolerance occurs by repeated experience with same. The scenario training method gives them this experience.

There is no difference between the chemical nature of the adrenaline that goes into their bloodstreams in a fight scenario and that of the adrenaline that will be introduced into their bloodstreams in an actual assault. If the fighter has had the adrenal experience in training and learned to control it there, he or she will be able to control it much better in an actual attack.

The scenario training method is effective because it faithfully replicates the most significant characteristics of every real combat situation: adrenal stress and how the fighter handles it.

PROPER RESPONSE TO ADRENAL
STRESS CAN BE LEARNED

Some people may think that they could never learn to remain calm when threatened or attacked. But such people simply have not had the opportunity to discover their true inner power, which adrenaline helps actualize.

Everyone can learn to improve their response to the adrenal stress of an attack very significantly, just as surely as people can learn to drive in city traffic. Scenario-based adrenal stress training conditions fighters to adrenaline so that they do not become overpowered by it and thus choke. *In addition,* it replaces this choke response with the attack response. The counterattack becomes instantaneous and full-force, as the adrenal force is channeled into the execution of effective technique (most particularly, striking technique). In this way, muscular memory is also established.

In the greater sense, because we are all made of the same clay, anyone can achieve this triumph over fear.

If you doubt this, consider this reality. When you are driving your car in normal traffic, you are routinely making life-and-death decisions. Usually, you just don't think about it this way, precisely because you are simply used to the stress of city driving. However, it is a fact that when you pull out across traffic you are judging the speed and distance of the oncoming car, and, though you don't give it much thought, you are betting your life, and often other people's lives, on your calculation that you can make it. However, a glance in the rearview mirror will tell you that the oncoming car crossed the intersection just a handful of seconds after you did. But, of course, this is no problem, because this is just like you "planned" it.

On a deeper level of your mind, you are aware of the actual physics of this driving situation. If you misjudge it by only four or five seconds, there will be a crash and you could be killed, crippled, or paralyzed. Still, you don't choke up thinking about this potential, because you are used to this situation. You have done it before. In your mind, *you have already made it* before you ever decide to pull out across the intersection.

Now, while I have this image in your mind, let me add that if you can face the guy coming at you with the tire iron with this same mind-set—that you have already made it—it will be much more likely that you will make it. (Read that again and think about it.) The central point here is that if you can get used to driving in city traffic you can get used to being woofed on or attacked, too. It chiefly depends on having some previous experience with the activity.

Can you remember the first time you got your driver's license and had to pull out across traffic? You were a lot more cautious, and it was all much more frightening. You were much more cognizant of the risks. Further, your perception of that risk affected your physical driving behavior. Consider how short a time it was before you became acclimated to this stress such that now that risk actually seems like an abstract thought.

Indeed, some people will eat, talk on their cellular phones, and tune the radio while merging onto a crowded freeway at 70 miles an hour. Most Aborigines in the Australian outback probably couldn't do this. Do you think it's because an Aborigine doesn't have the "courage" of our cellular phone user?

No, it's because these Aborigines don't have freeways and cars, so they haven't had a chance to get used to this form of stress or to learn the "simple" techniques of driving. But just as any Australian Aborigine can learn to drive on the freeway, any one of us can learn to deal much better with the adrenal stress of a combat situation and thus learn to defend himself much better. Individuals vary in many respects; indeed, this is the essence of the concept of "individual." But on the most fundamental level, we are all, indeed, made of the same clay.

ALL CRUELTY COMES FROM WEAKNESS

When people feel powerless, they feel weak and are afraid. Experiencing this fear, they either hide out, do some maiming and killing to show that they really aren't powerless and afraid, or, hopefully, choose to simply recognize and then begin to overcome their fear.

The typical case of the "hide out" personality is the bully who, every so often, has to have a drink or two and then find a victim to beat up or rape, so as to temporarily relieve his feeling of powerlessness, fear, and self-hatred. Then he can go hide out some more until that internal discord must be released again.

The most extreme example of the "powerless and

fearful" syndrome is people who plant a time bomb in a crowded building to do some killing and maiming in order to demonstrate that they are not powerless or afraid. They also are driven to show in dramatic and public fashion (though they intend to remain anonymous) that they just won't "take it" (whatever, in their own twisted minds, they have convinced themselves "it" is).

On the other hand, let us consider an extreme example of the better side of the human spirit, the vision of an individual who has recognized and dramatically overcome his fears. A story that comes to my mind is that of a priest who placed his body between the submachine guns of Nazi killers and their next intended victims as a shield.

Did he think the Nazis wouldn't shoot a priest? Wasn't he afraid to die as the 9mm bullets ripped through his body, as he had seen happen to others? Was his an act of lunacy or courage?

While a belief in "religion" has not been granted me, I submit that it was not an act of lunacy but an act of the most remarkable courage, made possible only by an actualization of the man's capacity for human compassion and empathy. This is what provided him with such strength. Apparently, in the face of such strength, even the Nazi killers somehow feared firing.

Also, I guess that priest was definitely having a lucky day.

· · · · ·

So why do I bring all this up? Because as violent as our modern world has become, and knowing that out of every hundred people we might train, at least two or three are later attacked, I believe that having overcome fear itself is just as valuable to these people in their daily lives as was the ability to overcome their assailant physically.

No such overcoming of fear is ever complete for anyone, of course. A complete transcendence of fear might even be termed a "psychopathology" itself, just as the priest's behavior when confronted with the Nazis might be seen as "crazy or irrational."

But it is clear to me that as we recognize and deal with our fear, we enlarge ourselves spiritually. We thus find it easier to be happier in our lives because we are less likely to allow the problems, frustrations, and discord surrounding our lives to become a discord within *ourselves*.

When we overcome fear it becomes possible to meet the world's everyday challenges (as well as its dangers) with a more relaxed and less fearful mind. We become less reactive and thus more free in our ability to make our own decisions about how we will act and how we will feel about our actions.

Physical violence, which is no more than being forced to deal with the extreme fear and discord in others, becomes easier to understand and thus to deal with effectively because we are neither denying its reality or being controlled by our own fear of it.

Now, my dear old dad used to say, "Son, you got to have something in your belly and a roof over your head before you can even think like that."

And, as was so often the case, he was quite right.

Now, here's what I say.

In facing and then moving toward overcoming our fear, any fear—the fear of assault; the fear of losing our job, our mate, our health; the fear of being afraid or alone; or that fear we all share and which is an inevitable certainty for us all, the fear of *death itself*—we are feeding ourselves spiritually, and we are thus putting that roof over our heads and that nourishment in our spiritual "bellies," which allows us to "think like that."

Overcoming fear allows us to act less out of anger and fear and more from the greater part of being . . . and that part is our capacity for empathy and human compassion.

Stay alert people . . . and peace be with you.

About the Author

Peyton Quinn began his training in formal Asian martial arts systems in 1964, eventually achieving rank in karate, judo, and, later in life, aikido.

While he continues to respect and explore these and other martial systems, his "real world" experience (including working as a bouncer in "problem bars") has demonstrated to him that, for most people, Asian martial arts systems alone are simply incomplete preparation for an actual attack.

In 1990, Quinn and his ex-bouncer pal Mike Haynack formed the Rocky Mountain Combat Applications Training Center in Boulder, Colorado. The essence of the RMCAT training method is the authentic fight simulation involving an armored assailant whose modus operandi is faithful to that of the assailants and the bully types observed so many times by both Peyton and Mike in their bouncer and other security-related work. The armored assailant (Bulletman) allows the fighter to go flat out with full-power striking in an unpredictable, dynamic fight scenario. In short, the fighter learns to fight by fighting!